the simple path to health

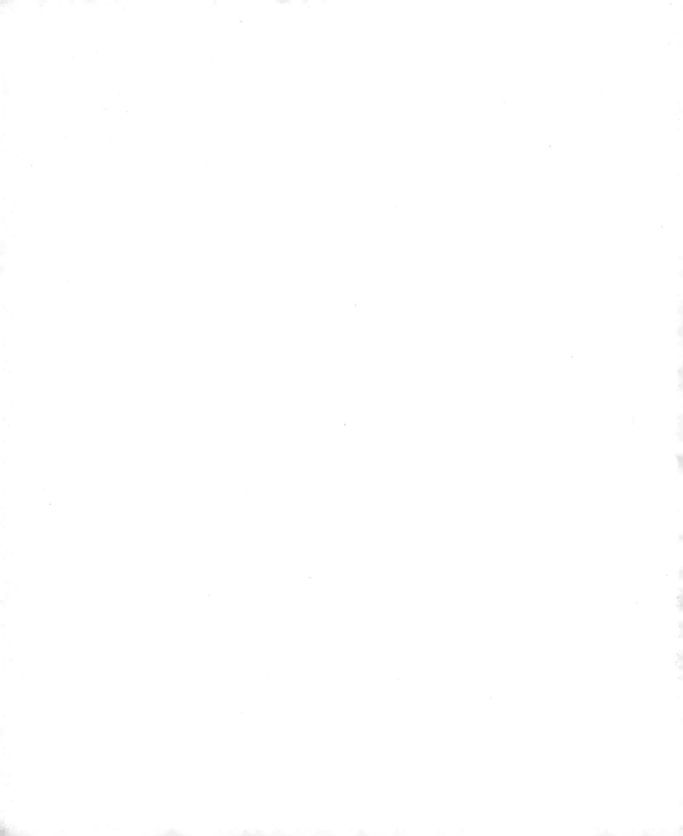

the simple path to health

A Guide to Oriental Nutrition and Well-Being

Kim Le, Ph.D.

RUDRA PRESS
PORTLAND OREGON

Rudra Press
PO Box 13390
Portland, Oregon 97213
Telephone: 503-235-0175
Telefax: 503-235-0909

Book design: Shannon Holt
Cover design: Bill Stanton & Shannon Holt
Cover illustration: Ana Capitaine
Interior illustrations: Hannah Bonner
Typography: Jeff Levin, Pendragon Graphics

This book is not intended to replace expert medical advice. The author and publisher urge you to verify the appropriateness of any procedure or exercise with your qualified health care professional. The author and publisher disclaim any liability or loss, personal or otherwise, resulting from the procedures and information in this book.

Library of Congress Cataloging-in-Publication Data

Le, Kim, 1949–
      The simple path to health : a guide to oriental nutrition and
well-being / Kim Le.
            p.   cm.
         ISBN 0-915801-62-0 (pbk.)
         1. Nutrition. 2. Medicine, Chinese. 3. Cookery, Chinese.
4. Diet therapy.   I. Title
RA784.L395   1996   96–3130
613'.0951—dc20   CIP

00 99 98 97   10 9 8 7 6 5 4 3 2

To my patients, associates, and friends, whom I have been able to serve over the years, and to those who seek a more fulfilling way of life.

Contents

CHARTS AND ILLUSTRATIONS

ACKNOWLEDGMENTS

i owe a great debt of gratitude to my parents for setting a bright example and instilling in me the necessity of living an honorable life in the service of God and mankind. I am also indebted to the many teachers who, over the years, have been kind enough to share their knowledge with me. I wish to express my deepest love and appreciation to my many patients, who have taught me so much about the art of healing. A special mention must be made in appreciation of Kassy Schloetzer for her painstaking efforts in capturing the spirit of this message and transcribing it into the original manuscript.

PREFACE

In my practice, I have found the dietary habits of my patients to be a major source of their problems. I have seen a lot of frustration and confusion and an almost hopeless look on the faces of many whom I begin treating. This is not because they don't want to eat well and stay healthy. It is because they lack the knowledge of the relationship of food and its preparation to the maintenance of health and a healthy state of mind.

Nineteen years ago, I qualified for a healing program at Ephrata Community Hospital in Pennsylvania. I was shocked and disappointed when everywhere I went I observed people suffering from many diseases, all mostly caused by a poor diet. Unlike here, hospitals in South Vietnam, where I grew up, are mostly reserved for military purposes. I was dismayed when I realized that, while in other countries people are fighting for freedom and dying because of war, here people are fighting for their lives and dying because of what they have chosen to put into their mouths.

This has concerned me deeply enough to be the subject of much contemplation in my spare time, as I pondered why this was the case and how it could be rectified. I was continually inspired, however, that in spite of a lack of knowledge, patients always showed a willingness and openness to make comprehensive changes and improvements, addressing the needs of the body, mind, and spirit as a unified experience.

I have been motivated to write this book not because I am a writer, but because the human drama within which I operate has presented an opportunity for me to fill a pressing need to supply answers to some very important questions. I wanted to make life easier for those who are seriously trying to improve their health and are excited by the promise of an opening of their awareness. I welcome this opportunity to assist you in your quest for well-being. For myself I have already been blessed in my healing work by being able to fulfill my lifelong dream of helping people and by being able to express fully the love and care I feel for those who have put their faith and trust in me.

Thank you again for allowing me this opportunity to share with you.

introduction

Choosing the Simple Path to Health

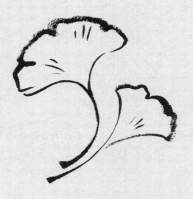

A PATH TO SELF-DISCOVERY

*i*n Oriental Medicine, health is seen as a balanced inter-relationship between body, mind, emotions, spirit, and the universe at large. This balanced state of health is viewed as our natural right. Illness is seen to be an unnatural state of imbalance that should not be tolerated. Bodily symptoms are treated as warning signals to right the wrongs we have brought upon ourselves through foods we ingest, attitudes we hold, and stressful lifestyles. In the Oriental view, if we live by nature's laws, we have a much better chance to live long, creative, and rewarding lives.

Your body is continually trying to balance itself in the face of constant stimulation from many sources—the environment, other people, your mind and spirit, and the cosmos. All your activities have an impact on this "balancing act." From this standpoint, there is no *final* place where you can rest in perfect health. As long as you are interacting with your environment, then your physical, emotional, and spiritual effort for balance will also continue. The dynamics of life that keep you continually struggling for balance also keep you growing and evolving. This is as it should be.

It is your job to keep the body in balance so that you can remain centered and healthy. This may take some reading, some study, and some use of your intuition. Many changes will be right for you that may not be right for others. Seeking across-the-board cure-alls is never fruitful.

This manual was written to help guide you along a simple path to self-discovery. It is designed to deepen your understanding of your body and your life, while giving you the courage to overcome obstacles on the road to wholistic well-being. I hope this will not just be another cook-book sitting on your shelf. By the same token, I know it does not contain answers to all the questions you may have. I hope it is valuable as a tool to guide you to a new state, along with many other tools you will acquire along your path. It may take you some time to refine your knowledge, but the process will be a joyful one bringing you the happiness of con-tinued vitality.

LISTENING TO THE SIGNALS OF NATURE

For those who have never been exposed to the foundations of wholis-tic medicine, some commonly held beliefs may have to be overcome. The most important one is the idea that when you become sick and tired, you have somehow been "victimized" by poor health. In most cases, you have simply been a victim of self-abuse. During my past twenty years in the healing profession, I have carefully observed the patterns of physical, emotional, and mental imbalances in each of my patients. It has become apparent from my observations that these symptoms are linked to the foods we consume and the lifestyles we choose to live.

Most treatments received for illnesses are symptomatic in nature, leaving the root of the problem untreated. I have concluded that we cre-ate illness, illness does not create itself. Only when we stop blaming external reasons and turn inward and look deeply into ourselves do we realize that disease is not manifested from thin air. Through this understanding we can begin to change ourselves, whether it is lifestyle, diet, way of thinking, or even our motivation for living.

In Western medicine, most treatment is tailored to analysis of the symptoms of a specific organ or area of the body, rather then a wholistic or preventive approach. In my practice, the primary focus is to treat the body, mind, and emotions of each patient. By this I mean learning to listen to the signals the body sends to let you know that you are off center. It is the nature of the body to give this direct feedback about our state of well-being.

Unfortunately, we're usually not taught to regard physical discomfort as an indication that we need to make changes in our physical, emotional, or spiritual life. We perpetuate living patterns and imbalances in our systems that deteriorate our health over a long period of time. All of this can be avoided by simply heeding the warning signals that nature provides and then following through on making needed changes. As soon as you notice that you are feeling tired all the time, that the simplest of life's situations are confusing you, or that you are experiencing a lack of motivation, you should tell yourself that it is time to turn your attention to your physical well-being. Accept the idea that your body will respond in a self-healing manner when you treat it well. The sooner you begin to heed warning signals, the sooner you will begin to heal.

Food is one of the main sources of energy and healing. In order to prepare a proper diet for yourself—one suitable to your present health, age, lifestyle, career situation, and emotional state—you need to understand your relationship to the ever-changing dynamics of the universe. Toward this endeavor, I am going to discuss how to balance your health and emotions by understanding the energy flow of your body and learning how to use and cook food according to universal laws.

Diet is a common contributor toward many illnesses in the majority of the patients I have seen. When a patient asks me, "Doctor, what can I do to improve my health?" my most common answer is, "Change your diet and your way of living!" The thousands of dollars you can save in doctor and hospital bills by simply eating and living in a healthy manner would astound you.

While eating right sounds simple, it is easier said than done. I'm sure you have attempted to diet at some time in your life and found it to be quite difficult. But over the long term, unless you embrace and adhere to a proper, nutritious diet, you will ultimately suffer the severe consequences of poor health. Remember, there is no free lunch. You can either pay the doctors and hospitals for them to treat your illnesses, or you can make an effort to eat properly and enjoy good health both now and later. The choice is yours.

There is no one best food for everyone. Diet should be tailored to each individual's needs. Some need food to detoxify, others need food to build up strength. Many need both. As we learn more about food and the therapeutic as well as energy-supplying properties it has, we will know when we need to change to different foods to keep ourselves balanced. In this way, we can fully utilize food as a tool for nourishment and health.

WHOLISTIC APPROACH TO TREATMENT

In general, traditional Chinese medicine has wholistic foundations and thus views all the organs as interdependent components of the whole. Isolating an organ and analyzing its malfunction is antithetical to this approach to the body. Furthermore, the organs are considered to go beyond their physiological functions and are seen to also serve as receptors and transmitters of cosmic energy.

We can use the lungs as an example. Western medicine teaches us that the lungs are the organs of respiration, through which the body is able to inhale oxygen and exhale carbon dioxide. Traditional Chinese medicine does not stop at this physical description. It teaches us that the lungs also play an important role in the production of protective Qi, known as Wei Qi. (Qi, or life force, is discussed in the next section of this book.) The lungs take the Qi from Heaven in the form of breath and distribute it to the entire body. At the same time, the lungs perform the delicate function of standing guard against the invasion of negative energies (germs, pollutants, etc.) which can deplete this protective Qi. Through exhalation, the lungs expel imbalancing forces originating in other parts of the body. The lungs also distribute liquids to the skin through the control of liquid metabolism; this is why patients suffering from asthma, bronchitis, sinus problems, and allergies usually have very dry skin.

When someone experiences grief, it will often manifest in the lungs as coughing or chest pain and the skin will feel excessively wet or dry. Since the lungs are also closely related to the colon, this grief can cause constipation or diarrhea. Conversely, if a problem originates in the colon, as in the case of too much toxicity, it may affect the lungs and manifest as sneezing, sinus problems, or allergies.

Based on the above, diseases can bee seen to originate in two ways: (1) as a result of reactions to outside forces that deplete the body's ability to protect itself and (2) as a result of unbalanced forces within the physical body that also cause a breakdown in its coping mechanism. In one case, the protective capacity of the lungs has been weakened by grief and has eventually affected the colon. In the other, a bad diet has caused excessive toxicity in the colon and has led to a diminishing of the lungs' ability to protect the Qi.

A logical consequence of the wholistic approach to the body is that dysfunction can be diagnosed by a healer as originating from any one of the three aspects of the entire system—the body, the mind, or the emotions. More importantly, no matter which aspect is considered to be the source of the problem, any recommendations to the patient will contain advice on how to address the needs of all three aspects of body, mind, and emotions.

For example, it is foolish to think you can drink one glass of milk a day or take calcium supplements to strengthen your bones. The body works as a whole, and when there is a malfunction somewhere, the whole body (body/mind/emotions) must be taken into careful consideration. A glass of milk will only cause more mucus in the system, and a tablet of calcium will only add to the burden of the liver. In order to increase the absorption of invaluable substances from the foods you consume each day, you must adjust your diet, and work to rid yourself of the fears and anxieties that can interfere with your body's utilization of the nutrients it needs to build strength. Maintaining a healthy body is a job that requires work each and every day. A handful of vitamins will never take the place of the loving attention you reap upon your magnificent machine on a daily basis.

the balance of life

An Overview of Oriental Philosophy

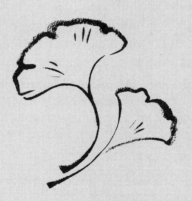

YIN/YANG UNDERSTANDING

through careful observation of the changes and flow of nature, ancient oriental thinkers and healers developed a deep understanding of life. They saw that in its essence, life is a process involving a polarity of forces which interact inextricably to express themselves in a variety of forms. But this variety exists within the boundaries of a unified whole, as changeless as its expression is ever-changing. From this recognition, the Yin/Yang theory developed, wherein the two polar forces were named Yin and Yang. The following symbol evolved to express the basic concepts imbedded in the theory.

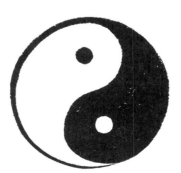

To embrace the meaning of the symbol is to understand that it represents the vibratory nature of all manifest phenomena, created by the interaction of opposing yet complementary forces—the positive and negative, the aggressive and receptive, the masculine and feminine—all existing to encourage balance in the unfolding of life.

The circle, enclosing what appears to be two dolphins playing, represents the cosmic oneness within which these forces operate—the unity of life. What is interesting and significant is that the white dolphin has a black eye and the black dolphin has a white eye; the symbology being that if white is soft and black is hard, there is neither a total softness nor a total hardness—each has within itself a perception or an inlet to its opposite. This presence of opposite aspects also suggests the constant movement of yin and yang, one into the other, stimulated by the physical laws of attraction and repulsion. This movement is what guarantees that change, growth, and evolution will occur as part of the life process.

Human beings are inextricably part of the whole of nature and as such are themselves an expression of the interplay of forces, of Yin and Yang. Our bodies, our breath, the way we work, play, and think—all originate from and manifest the interaction of these two forces. Accepting this, the principles of Yin/Yang theory encourage a wholistic view of life and suggest it can be lived as a work of art.

By understanding the applications of Yin/Yang theory to all aspects of life, a person can achieve the balance so essential to a sense of well-being. Life's activities are never isolated from each other; by contemplating the interaction of Yin/Yang forces within us, we can learn to express ourselves, take care of our bodies, and nourish ourselves in a balanced way.

To guide us in applying Yin/Yang theory to the dynamics of our lives, the "Seven Universal Principles" evolved:

1. **There is infinite variety in the world, but there is only one Source.** God, as the Source, is energy whose nature is a balanced interplay of creation and withdrawal; this energy expresses itself as the variety of manifestation in the universe. Knowing this, we see ourselves as part of the self-expressive, creative energy of God, and know we are guided toward our own self-expression by this force.

2. **Everything changes.** Everything is in continuous flow and change. Knowing this we understand that we are part of a process. We understand that our activities are not an end in themselves. We're encouraged to embrace change as an opportunity for growth, understanding, and for fulfilling our destiny.

3. **Everything interrelates with everything else.** Everything is part of an enormous cosmic system that thrives on co-operation and a balance of forces. Knowing this keeps us conscious of the whole and encourages us to act for the benefit of the whole. From this follows the recognition that when we put negative energy into the process, we ultimately affect our own progress. This also encourages us to be willing to look into something seemingly disastrous and see the good behind it, knowing that it is only temporary.

4. **No two things are identical.** Each of us has something unique to offer. This knowledge encourages us not to be afraid to have a different idea, to remember that variety is necessary for the whole color of the garden. We can only fulfill our own true nature. With this in mind, however, we must also remember that we are still a part of God's infinite life form.

5. **What has a front has a back.** This relates to our concept of cause and effect. What you set in motion is going to unfold as your life. This knowledge should encourage us to have a positive outlook in all our endeavors so that what we manifest from our thoughts and activities will enhance our well-being.

6. **The bigger the front, the bigger the back.** The more powerful the beginning, the more powerful the ending. This relates to the power behind our dynamic choices and should guide us to put the greatest energy to those tasks that we know will create the greatest good.

7. **What has a beginning has an end.** Anything that we set in motion will have an outcome. We reap experiences commensurate with the seeds that we plant, and we cannot avoid that outcome. This knowledge encourages us to set our activities in motion with clarity of thought and purpose. This knowledge also lets us accept graciously that all things, events, and even our bodies will pass.

The Yin / Yang theory and the seven universal principles make up the foundation of oriental medicine and its approach to health and healing, just as the scientific principles and the laws of physics are the basis of Western modern medicine. Throughout this book, the oriental approach is the basis for understanding body processes, for diagnosing illnesses, for selecting balancing foods to eat, and for approaching a state of well-being. Since in this theory of ebb and flow, life is seen as a process, no single answer is correct for everyone, nor for the same person at different times. The pursuit of health thus becomes a path of living in balance with ourselves and all of nature.

THE VITAL FORCE—QI

Traditional Chinese medicine teaches that all living forms contain a life force called "Qi". It is the physical energy of life which expresses itself through the principles of Yin and Yang. Qi is the vital force which gives life to all animate bodies. Many people have been introduced to the concept of Qi through the study of T'ai Chi, Qi Gong, or some other martial art. Yet Qi is a mystery; it is formless, invisible, and difficult to measure and prove, although it can be palpably experienced and its effects observed. Qi can be simply thought of as an electromagnetic force field that keeps us "grounded" to the earth and which when condensed brings matter into form.

Qi is the force which gives movement and heat to life. Our breath— each inhalation and exhalation—is moved by Qi. The wind and the tides are the action of Qi. When Qi is light it flows freely. When Qi is blocked, contracted, or stagnant, it becomes heavy and oppressive. Health and well-being are the manifestation of Qi freely flowing through our bodies. Illness results when Qi becomes blocked, stagnant, or out of balance. Death is the manifestation of Qi leaving our bodies.

In the Oriental view, Qi is vital to all existence and is a most precious commodity which is enhanced by mastering the art of living. It cannot be bottled and sold in a jar. Only a raising of consciousness through the daily practice of healthy living habits will strengthen it. In human beings, this life force is maintained and can be enhanced by two main activities: (1) breathing and (2) food intake.

Throughout this guidebook there are frequent references to the different types of Qi, and all efforts are focused on how to develop this vital force. It is hoped that this focus will help you embrace the essence of Qi and strengthen it in your daily life. Mastering the art of living in this way will help you unfold the mystery of eternity.

The Law of the Five Elements

A further unfolding of the Oriental medicine model is the concept that the material world is composed of the basic elements wood, fire, earth, metal, and water. These have an innate interdependence and inter-restraint whereby they are held in a state of constant motion and change. The Five Elements represent different levels of the same phenomenon; if you refer to one element, you refer to all because of their interrelationship. This is the Law of the Five Elements.

Each element denotes a category of related functions and qualities. These qualities contain the opposites of production and destruction, stimulation and inhibition. To understand these qualities and their relationships to each other is to begin to understand the process of change and manifestation in life; thus we begin to understand the complex nature of cause and effect. The table and diagram below outline these interrelationships.

ELEMENT	BASIC FUNCTIONS
Wood	Associates with active functions that are in a growing state.
Fire	Designates functions that have reached a maximal state of activity and are about to begin to decline to a resting period.
Earth	Designates balance or neutrality.
Metal	Represents functions in a declining state.
Water	Represents functions that have reached a maximal state of rest and are about to change the direction of their activity.

One essential characteristic of the Five Elements is production. In this regard, each element has two purposes—to produce and to be produced. Wood produces fire, fire produces earth, earth produces metal,

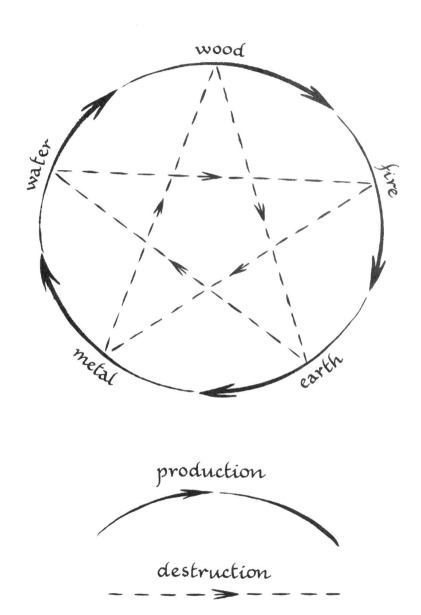

PRODUCTION/DESTRUCTION OF THE FIVE ELEMENTS

metal produces water, and water produces wood. "Produce" implies to nourish, maintain, assist, stimulate. For example, metal produces water; metal is the "mother" of water; water produces wood; wood is the "son" of water. The same applies to the other elements:

ELEMENT	ELEMENT ACTED UPON IN PRODUCTION
Wood	Fire
Fire	Earth
Earth	Metal
Metal	Water
Water	Wood

The second essential quality of the Five Elements is destruction. Wood destroys earth, earth destroys water, water destroys fire, fire destroys metal, and metal destroys wood. "Destroy" implies to defeat, oppress, prevent, inhibit. For example, wood uses its energies to restrain earth, which in turn restrains water. Thus, each element presents the double aspect of destroying and being destroyed.

ELEMENT	ELEMENT ACTED UPON IN DESTRUCTION
Wood	Earth
Earth	Water
Water	Fire
Fire	Metal
Metal	Wood

Each element has a corresponding season, environmental factor, phase of growth and development, color, taste, and direction. The chart titled "The Five Elements and the Six Categories of Nature" shows these relationships. As we progress through this book, you'll learn about these correspondences and how they apply to our bodies, its organs, its vital processes, and to the food we eat.

THE FIVE ELEMENTS AND THE SIX CATEGORIES OF NATURE

Element	Season	Environmental Factor	Growth & Development	Color	Taste	Direction
Wood	Spring	Wind	Germination	Green	Sour	East
Fire	Summer	Heat	Growth	Red	Bitter	South
Earth	Late summer	Dampness	Transformation	Yellow	Sweet	Middle
Metal	Autumn	Dryness	Reaping	White	Pungent	West
Water	Winter	Cold	Storing	Black	Salty	North

We've now covered basic elements in the Oriental view of life and phenomena. I've tried to present the material simply, without losing the essential teaching. It is not my goal to have you become Chinese philosophers, Rather, my hope is that you will gain insight into the foundations from which Oriental medicine sprang and will be inspired to a more wholistic view so that you can make practical and lasting changes in your daily life. In the next section, we'll expand on these principles to further understand the traditional Chinese medicine approach to the human body system and its diagnosis and treatment.

the human body system

A Chinese Medicine View of the Body

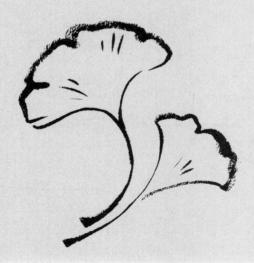

QI IN THE HUMAN BODY

traditional Chinese medicine views mankind as the union of the finest essence energy of Heaven and Earth. The first breath we take at birth is energy that connects us with our origin and thrusts us onto the Wheel of Life to take advantage of the opportunities life presents to grow and evolve. In this view, the body is considered a divine instrument, completely connected and permeated with the field of energy which is all of life. The body is made up of the same Five Elements and is subject to the laws of the polar yin and yang that are present in nature. Qi, the vital force of life, is the vital force which sustains the body. The body is understood to be permeated with an energetic network through which Qi flows and is stored.

The energy network of the human body is made up of a system of channels and meridians. These are conduits of energy flow, both on the surface and the deep interior of the body. Twelve major meridians correspond with the twelve major organ systems of the body. (These will be discussed in a later section.) The meridians act as "rivers" of energy running through the organ systems and extending to other parts of the body. They irrigate the organ systems and bring vitality to their functions. In addition to the twelve major meridian "rivers", there are eight extraordinary channels which store and feed energy into the twelve organ meridians. These act as "reservoirs" of energy.

The meridians and extraordinary channels, however, are not limited in their influence to the organ system for which they are named. They are also responsible for physiological functions in other parts of the body to which they extend. For example, the liver meridian starts inside the big toe, travels up past the genital area, past the liver, up the breast to the throat, the eyes, and then to the top of the head. An Oriental practitioner will often understand many eye problems to be symptomatic of a liver dysfunction or a blockage of flow in the liver meridian. In oriental medicine, illness and its resulting symptoms are understood to be results of imbalances or blockages of the flow of Qi through the channels, and diagnosis is achieved through a holistic understanding of this energy mechanism.

The human body receives its Qi from two primary sources. Ancestral Qi (also referred to as Kidney Qi or Congenital Qi) is inherited from the chromosomes in the sperm and ovum of our parents. Ancestral Qi is the union of the masculine and feminine essences of our ancestors and is stored in our glands, hormones, and kidneys. This Qi is considered a prenatal Qi. It is unchangeable. We receive only what has been given to us and store it or use it in our own reproductive processes.

Acquired Qi, or postnatal Qi, is the body's second major source of energy. We obtain it from the essence of food and air. Unlike Ancestral Qi, we do have the ability to strengthen the Qi in our bodies through Acquired Qi, as we have control over our food intake and to some extent our breathing. We can make sure that we eat only those foods that will contribute to the maintenance of our well-being, and we can affect the air we breathe by keeping our environment as clean and pure as possible. If we engage in these activities with mindfulness, we will maintain a healthy balance between the yin and yang forces within us and assure ourselves the vibrancy of strong Qi.

Human energy is further differentiated into a number of different types. *Wei Qi* is the protective energy which forms a layer over the surface of the body, guarding the body from disruption and intrusion. *Ying Qi* is the nourishing energy which flows within the energy meridians. The functions, cycles, and flow of these two energies will be discussed in detail in the next sections. Other forms of Qi briefly referred to are Essential Qi and *Zong Qi*. Essential Qi is formed in the chest to nourish the heart and lungs and promote their functions of regulating the blood vessels and performing respiration. Zong Qi is the combination of Acquired Qi and the essence energy of food. All of these forms of Qi are derived from the combined essence of food, air, and the inherited Ancestral Qi.

External energies in the environment and the food that we eat continually affect the electromagnetic field of the human body system and the flow of Qi. We are in a constant state of exchange with our environment through our food intake and breathing. Thus, we can see how our selection and preparation of food and our choice of lifestyle have a powerful influence on our health and well being. In fact, careful attention to these things is the fundamental way in which we can maintain some control over our own destinies.

The most important way in which food contributes to strong Qi, and thus our health, is through the effect it has on our immune system and the protective Wei Qi. Eating foods which are in balance with your body's constitution and which harmonize the yin and yang forces within the body, will serve to strengthen your Qi. By strengthening the Wei Qi, food can serve as a source of protection from outside invasions that can weaken the body's defense mechanisms. Eating nutritious food will give us the psychological as well as physical strength to cope with life's stresses and strains.

Needless to say, we are living in a world where illnesses such as AIDS, cancer, and heart disease threaten our existence every day. We cannot avoid being in the world, but we can control our health practices and minimize these threats if we are conscious about what we feed our bodies. By consciously staying in tune with the natural laws that govern your body, and adjusting your diet and living habits to support and harmonize with its functions, you are able to take into your hands the care for your own health. In the next sections, I will explain the relationship of the natural laws to your own body's processes.

THE DEFENSIVE WEI QI— HOW IT WORKS

All forms of Qi aid the body's responses to its environment. Wei Qi energy, also known as the "defensive Qi," plays an important role in these responses. In the context of a nutritional guidebook it deserves particular attention because of its direct relationship to the transformation of food into defensive energy and the importance of this process in the eventual awakening of the latent spiritual energies within us. This section on the formation and function of Wei Qi energy will help you understand the importance of all forms of Qi in keeping the body fortified and alert to environmental conditions.

Wei Qi is a protective layer of energy covering the body just below the skin layer. It forms a protective shield which supplies us with information about our environment and guards against the entrance of negative outside forces and contaminants. The simple cross-section diagram following shows the relationship of Wei Qi energy to the skin, the principal meridian (with a yin and yang component), and the blood.

Food and breath are the ingredients from which Wei Qi energy is formed. We need food to survive, and we need breath to supply the energy to digest the food. Wei Qi is produced when these two ingredients are combined, transformed into essence energy, and then channeled by the other organs through a process known as The Five Levels of Purification. We will discuss this process in detail later.

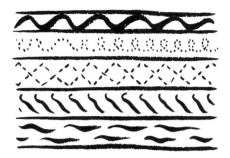

skin

wei chi

combination of zong and wei chi

combination of zong chi and principal meridians

blood

In the purification process, the essences of food and air are transformed into Wei Qi in the liver. While we sleep Wei Qi is transformed into steam. Because steam rises, the Wei Qi energy moves upward through the thorax, neck, and face and is stored in the outer cantus of the eyes. Remember that in our earlier discussion, we pointed out that the liver meridian passes through the eyes.

By the time we get up in the morning, Wei Qi energy is ready to go to work. Our natural instincts cause us to rub our eyes or to blink a lot in the process of waking up. This stimulates the Wei Qi energy to travel outward through the capillaries to all parts of the skin, where it serves as "protective Qi." It circulates so rapidly that it is also frequently referred to as "mobile energy" because it "mobilizes" the body's defense mechanisms. It places the body in a state of immediate preparedness to meet all the demands of everyday life, both cosmic (sun, wind, storms) and biophysical (negative emotions, wrong food).

Wei Qi energy plays a significant role in informing us of changes in our environment or in the flow of energy. When it is drafty or you are exposed to negative energy, you may sneeze or experience a chill. This is the result of Wei Qi reacting underneath the skin to inform you of changes. Most discomfort you feel throughout the day is Wei Qi energy serving as an early warning system to keep you alert to environmental conditions. It also rests in the tips of the toes and fingers to act in the same capacity. (For those studying acupuncture, Spleen 6 is another destination of Wei Qi energy because it is the connection point of the energies of the kidney, spleen, and liver.)

The movement of Wei Qi energy has a daytime cycle and a nighttime cycle. The nighttime cycle begins when we retire for the evening and decrease our need for defensive preparedness. At this point, as energy continues to pass through the purification process, the body's sensing mechanisms signal Wei Qi energy to begin concentrating in the liver. The nighttime cycle ends when Wei Qi is turned into steam and moves upward to rest in the outer cantus of the eyes.

As previously described, the daytime cycle is initiated when we blink or rub our eyes on rising in the morning. The Wei Qi energy that has been forming all night is immediately distributed throughout the body and stored under the skin. Subsequently, the body continues to create essence energy from food and breath through the process of the Five Levels of Purification, and Wei Qi energy is replenished throughout the active hours of your day.

All diseases must first penetrate Wei Qi's protective shield. Diseases can take hold in the body only when Wei Qi has become very weak because of system imbalances. Conversely, most conditions can be reversed by replenishing or strengthening Wei Qi through a combination of dietary adjustments, improved breathing techniques, and an appropriate amount of exercise to help release toxins.

Understanding the process of the formation and distribution of Wei Qi energy is a very important aspect of Oriental diagnosis. Through this understanding a practitioner can deduce where a patient may have become "stuck" at a certain level of purification or energy transformation. Usually this has occurred through poor dietary habits, poor breathing techniques, negative attitudes, or in many cases, a combination of all three.

I realize that these ideas are foreign to the Western concept of disease formation; however, they make up the basic knowledge underlying

Oriental healing and medicine. Acupuncture treatments are effective in that they can reactivate the powerful protective qualities of Wei Qi energy and thus encourage a release of system blockages and a restrengthening of the body's immune system. In this way, the body is not "healed from" a disease, but rather it is refortified to perform the "self-healing" functions made possible by the circulation and distribution of Wei Qi.

The saying of computer users, "garbage in, garbage out" certainly applies in the discussion of Wei Qi formation. In order to ensure the maintenance of strong Wei Qi, we must consume food that contains within it the highest essence energy possible and which is in harmony with nature and our own constitution. Eating junk foods or foods which are stripped of much of their natural essence will lead to a weakening of our own energy. When our supply of Wei Qi energy is depleted, we not only lose our instinctive ability to stay close to those activities which enhance our well-being, but our immune systems weaken and we become susceptible to all forms of sickness. Common sense tells us that we can expect no more from the efficient functioning of our immune systems than the care we put into them.

It is not surprising that a degeneration in the quality of food consumed by the average American and a lack of emphasis on the importance of practicing proper deep breathing techniques have been accompanied by the emergence of so many health problems that stem from a weakened immune system (AIDS, cancer, and heart disease, for example). In addition, millions of dollars are spent in laboratory research in an effort to discover cures for diseases that in many cases are simply the result of maintaining a poor diet over a long period of time. Individual efforts to study and practice wholistic health habits would go a long way toward reducing the burden of illness on society by regenerating the protective strength of Wei Qi energy.

THE ORGANS AND THE FIVE ELEMENTS

As part of nature, we carry within us the same material that makes up the earth and all other living entities. This is most clearly seen by the presence of the Five Elements in the different components of the body and the influence the elements have on the physio-spiritual functioning of the organs. For instance, the element of earth is contained in the flesh and skin; the element of water in the blood and mucus; the element of wood in bone; the element of fire in the warmth of the body; and the element of metal in the composition of the cells.

ELEMENT	PRESENCE IN THE BODY
Earth	Flesh and Skin
Water	Blood and Mucus
Wood	Bone
Fire	Body Heat
Metal	Cell Composition

All these are exchanging energy on a continual basis to cause a dynamic equilibrium that creates the forces of yin and yang to encourage forward motion and development. At a fundamental level, we are also subject to the same dynamic forces that result from the interrelationship of these elements. Thus the body's functions are a reflection of the broader universal principles.

Understanding the function of each organ is necessary in order to make adjustments to your diet that will contribute to an ongoing balance in your system. At the same time, we must remember that traditional Chinese medicine has holistic foundations and thus views all the organs as interdependent components of the whole. Isolating an organ in analyzing its malfunction is antithetical to this understanding of the body and its health needs. Furthermore, the organs are considered to go beyond their physiological functions to also serve as receptors and transmitters of cosmic energy.

Western medicine has been slow in recognizing the importance of this comprehensive approach, but its simple effectiveness cannot be denied. Oriental medicine embraces the body as a magnificent mechanism that is continually striving to stay in balance by compensating for emotional and spiritual responses to the environment. Each organ is seen as having a "door" through which excesses are manifested and released. By understanding these processes, we can assist rather than inhibit the body's amazing ability to heal itself. Keep this viewpoint in mind as you read the material on the function and significance of each organ.

Organs are designated into two categories: "Solid Organs" and "Hollow Organs." The Chinese word for "Solid Organs" is *Zang*. Solid organs are collectively known as yin channels. "Hollow Organs" are called *Fu* and are known as yang channels. Each of these organs is associated with one of the Five Elements and its functions. In addition to the solid organs and hollow organs, Chinese medicine describes a third category of "Extraordinary" organs which includes the brain and uterus. The following table shows the organ categories and their corresponding element.

ELEMENT	SOLID ORGAN: *ZANG* (Yin Channels)	HOLLOW ORGAN: *FU* (Yang Channels)
Wood	Liver	Gall Bladder
Fire	Heart	Triple Burner
	Pericardium	Small Intestine
Earth	Spleen	Stomach
Metal	Lung	Colon
Water	Kidney	Urinary Bladder

Each of the organs relates to each other organ in a way corresponding to the production/destruction diagram of the Five Elements presented earlier. Recall that "produce" implies to nourish, maintain, assist, stimulate; "destroy" implies to defeat, oppress, prevent, inhibit. These relationships between the organs are shown in the table below and the illustration which follows.

ORGAN	ORGAN ACTED UPON IN PRODUCTION	ORGAN ACTED UPON IN DESTRUCTION
Liver	Heart	Spleen
Heart	Spleen	Lung
Spleen	Lung	Kidney
Lung	Kidney	Liver
Kidney	Liver	Heart

This helps us understand the cyclical nature of the body processes and the flow of energy through the system. As we will see when we discuss the Five Levels of Purification, these production/destruction relationships govern the transformation of food and air into energy of the body.

In addition to organs, the Five Elements also have corresponding senses, tissues, and emotions. These will be discussed to a lesser extent in this guidebook; the chart below shows some of these classifications.

THE FIVE ELEMENTS AND THE CORRESPONDING FIVE BODY CATEGORIES

Five Elements	ZANG (Solid Organ)	FU (Hollow Organ)	Sense Organ	Body Tissue	Emotion
Wood	Liver	Gall bladder	Eye	Tendon	Anger
Fire	Heart	Sm. intestine	Tongue	Vessel	Joy
Earth	Spleen	Stomach	Mouth	Muscle	Meditation
Metal	Lung	Lg. intestine	Nose	Skin & hair	Grief & melancholy
Water	Kidney	Urinary bladder	Ear	Bone	Fright & fear

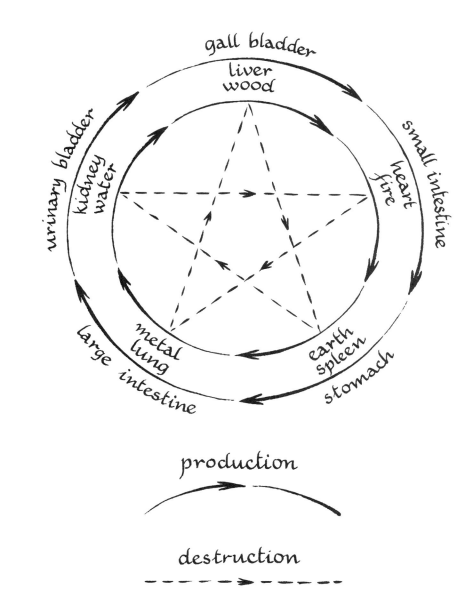

gall bladder

liver
wood

urinary bladder

kidney
water

small intestine

heart
fire

metal
lung

large intestine

earth
spleen

stomach

production

destruction

PRODUCTION/DESTRUCTION OF THE FIVE ELEMENTS
AND THEIR RELATED ORGANS

FUNCTION AND SIGNIFICANCE OF EACH ORGAN

LIVER

Description and Functions

The liver channel (meridian) starts inside the big toe, travels up past the genital area, past the liver, up the breast to the throat, the eyes, and then to the top of the head. The liver's main physiological functions are to clean, strengthen, and regulate the supply of blood to the body, thus maintaining potency for the flow of Qi. It also controls the sinews, muscles, and joints, and regulates the functioning of the nervous system. It is considered the "General" within the organism because it is in charge of the body's defense strategy. This strategy is carried out by the storing and releasing of Wei Qi energy, which we have described earlier as the defense energy of the body. The liver has the following corresponding properties and aspects:

PROPERTY	ASPECT
Emotion	Anger
Body Fluid	Tears
Season	Spring
Environmental Factor	Wind
Phase of Growth	Germination
Color	Green
Taste	Sour
Direction	East
Healing Sound	SHU

Liver Imbalance

The liver most often suffers from conditions of excess. These are usually rooted in emotional imbalance, build-up and suppression of anger, frustration, fear, depression, irritability, or stress. The imbalances of excess are also exacerbated by over consumption of alcohol, cigarettes, and junk foods.

If a person often becomes angry and attempts to suppress the anger, storing it rather than releasing it, the liver Qi can rebel. Symptoms will manifest along the liver meridian through headaches, sore breasts, a sensation of a lump in the throat, or blurry eyes. If the condition is prolonged without being treated, the liver Qi eventually invades the spleen and there can be digestive problems such as vomiting, nausea, acid eructation, heartburn, abdominal distention, flatulence, or diarrhea. Advanced cases of liver imbalances may suffer from chronic headaches, dizziness, redness of the face and eyes, blurred vision, glaucoma, soft nails, or a chronic or recurring sore throat.

The first obvious liver imbalance signs may be one or several of the following:

- redness in the eyes

- a throbbing headache, usually on the top of the head

- a red tongue with a yellow coating

- the voice may project too loudly or coarsely

- skin with a light yellow or light green color

- pulse that is wiry and chorded

- irritability and impatience

- teariness (The liver often causes the formation of tears to "wash away" excessive anger.)

- Painful or difficult menstrual cycle (blood dark red, scanty, and malodorous and an experience of cramping and bad temper).

- sore throat

- skin problems

If an excessive liver condition is not treated properly and persists, further symptoms may develop:

- Constipation .

- Hemorrhoids

- Toxic blood and a toxic lymphatic system resulting from chronic constipation

Dreams

According to the *Nei Ching*, an ancient Chinese textbook, exhaustion of liver energy often manifests in dreams of mushrooms or a sensation of lying under a tree and not daring to get up. The *Ling Shu*, another ancient text, instructs that with a liver energy deficiency, one may dream of a tree in a mountain forest.

Cleansing the Liver

An initial "cleaning" of the liver to rid built-up toxins will often help begin the process of restoring balance to this organ system. The following remedies can assist in cleansing the liver; appropriate caution and moderation, however, should always be exercised. They are not offered in the spirit of a quick cure.

1. 1 tbsp. olive oil
   $\frac{1}{2}$ cup pure apple cider vinegar or $\frac{1}{2}$ lemon
   1 cup of warm distilled water

   Mix and drink in the morning on an empty stomach for a week. If the remedy makes you feel weak or sick, the cleansing may be happening too fast. In this case, reduce the frequency to once every other day and add steamed vegetables to your diet to maintain your strength as you are cleansing.

2. Cook $\frac{1}{2}$ cup of mung beans in 4 cups of water in a slow cooker overnight. Drink this juice and eat the mung beans. Repeat every other day for two weeks. Those who are anemic should check with their acupuncturist or physician first.

3. Eat corn on the cob and save the corn silk. You may put the corn silk in the sun to dry for later use. Make corn silk tea and drink throughout the day.

As you begin a cleansing process, please be aware that it takes a long period of abusing your body with the wrong food to upset your emotions and damage your liver. It will naturally take a long period of time to heal it by adhering to a balanced diet. Sometimes when you feel you have found an answer to your problem, you may go to extremes in trying to effect a "quick cure." You may also be tempted to seek external solutions such as taking mega doses of vitamins, trying fad diets, or using "miracle" herbs. This will have the opposite effect of what you desire, since they will add to the burden on your liver. Such cures will only delay your return to optimum health.

Diet is not always the only answer. Changing any troubling or uncomfortable circumstances, being able to talk to a friend who is a good listener, and receiving acupuncture treatments regularly will help the "will-to-be" become stronger and reestablish the flow of Qi through the entire body. To obtain the most long-lasting, effective results, it is best to consult your acupuncturist or a physician who has a background in Chinese medicine and will take into consideration your emotional and mental problems as well as your physical condition.

HEART

The heart meridian is related to the small intestine and opens onto the tongue. The main physiological functions of the heart are to direct the working of the blood vessels and pulses. The heart is considered the sovereign ruler ("King") of the body because it is the residence of the directing energy called "Shen"—the spirit or divine energy of the individual. Shen participates in and regulates the activities of all spheres of being, including the facets of the personality. From the heart, this energy moves upward to the brain where it functions as the mind, and downward to the organs, where it functions as the balancing center of the entire organism. This is why it is often said that whatever we hold in our heart will be in our mind and result in the life that we lead. It is also said that the tongue is the mirror of the heart because the heart meridian opens onto the tongue. In fact, we all instinctively understand that talking is one way to relieve heartache. Following are the heart's properties and aspects:

PROPERTY	ASPECT
Emotion	Joy
Season	Summer
Environmental Factor	Heat
Phase of Growth	Growth
Color	Red
Taste	Bitter
Direction	South
Healing Sound	HU

Dreams

When the heart energy is out of balance, yang phenomena will appear in dreams. An overabundance of heart energy may manifest in a dream as laughing easily or seeing blazing flames. With an acute deficiency of heart energy, hills of ashes and gray mountains often appear.

PERICARDIUM

The pericardium is a protective membrane that surrounds the heart. It is the reservoir of energy entrusted to the individual at birth. It is the origin of joy and sadness and has two main functions: (1) to protect the heart sphere and (2) to maintain the order of its energy.

The pericardium is not regarded as an independent organ but as an attachment to the heart. It stands next to the heart as a guard would stand next to a king. In speaking of "heart failure," what actually occurs is the failure of the pericardium to protect the "king." For this reason, it is referred to as the "official ambassador" of the heart sphere.

SPLEEN

The primary function of the spleen is to control the transformation, distribution, and storage of nourishment and energy for the entire body. The spleen's physiological function is the regulation of blood volume. When referring to the spleen, it is understood in Chinese medicine that the activities of the pancreas are also included.

The spleen works in conjunction with the stomach to transform the liquid from food into energy and distribute it to the other organs of the body for absorption. It stores the nourishing energy of the body (Ying Qi) in the middle burner. The *Su Wen* says: "Food enters the stomach and the essence is driven off and passes through the spleen. The energy of the spleen transforms the essence, which then rises to the lungs."

The extension of the spleen energy is the flesh and its outward manifestation is the lips. It opens out to the mouth, and its sense organ is the tongue. The *Ling Shu* makes the following distinction: "If the energy of the heart is in harmony, the tongue may distinctly perceive the five flavors. If the energy of the spleen is in harmony, the tongue may perceive whether food is palatable."

The spleen is considered the most vital organ in spiritual growth because it receives direct energy from the sun and transforms it into energy that nourishes the entire body. It plays an essential role in the workings of the memory and the imagination. The quality of spleen energy directly influences the level of one's spiritual attainment. The properties and aspects of the spleen are:

PROPERTY	ASPECT
Emotion	Meditation, pondering, or reminiscence
Body Fluid	Saliva
Season	Late Summer
Environmental Factor	Dampness
Phase of Growth	Transformation
Color	Yellow
Taste	Sweet
Direction	Center Point or Middle

Spleen Imbalance

Traditional Chinese medicine considers the spleen to be the most vital organ in the body because it is able to transform food into a refined form that can nourish the whole body. Just as important, it simultaneously transforms thought into a form of energy that can nourish the spirit. Thus any spleen deficiency will have an immediate debilitating effect on both the physical and spiritual vitality of the entire organism.

Since the liver is responsible for controlling and checking the spleen energy, the quality and expression of the spleen energy is greatly dependent on the performance and purity of the liver energy. Lacking this purity, the entire body may then be left feeling very vulnerable owing to its inability to produce sufficient amounts of protective Wei Qi energy. Chronic loose stool or frequent diarrhea is a sign of spleen energy exhaustion.

A deficiency will not only make you feel physically depleted owing to a lack of nourishment but may also cause the formation of negative thought patterns that can lead to depression and personality dysfunction. In short, spleen deficiencies can seriously impair survival mechanisms and, ultimately, the promise of spiritual development.

Dreams

According to the *Nei Ching*, if the energy of the spleen is exhausted, one dreams that one lacks food and drink. One may also dream of erecting walls and buildings. The *Ling Shu* states that if the spleen energy is abundant, one dreams of chanting and playing music; yet one's body is heavy and one cannot rise. If acute deficiency of spleen energy exists, in one's dreams there appear hills and marshes, ruined buildings, and storms.

LUNGS

Western medicine teaches us that the lungs, which are situated in the thorax, are the organs of respiration through which the body is able to inhale oxygen and exhale carbon dioxide. Traditional Chinese medicine does not stop at this physical description. In addition, the lungs are related to the large intestine (colon) and the lung meridian opens out to the nose and the skin.

The lungs control breathing and the flow of Qi, the fundamental vital factors for sustaining life. They do this by taking the Qi from Heaven in the form of breath and distributing it to the entire body. At the same time, the lungs perform the delicate functions of standing guard against the invasion of negative energies which can deplete this protective Qi (germs, polluted air, bacteria, etc.) and expelling imbalancing forces originating in other parts of the body through exhalation.

Because the body depends on the lungs to maintain rhythmic order, they hold the office of "Minister" within the organism. When the breath and Qi are working harmoniously, the nourishing (Ying) and defensive (Wei) energies of the body and all other organs have the best chance of lining up in good working order. The lungs also play an important role in the production of protective Wei Qi. They affect the liver's functions in Wei Qi production, because the lung's opening to the skin is one of the eventual pathways of Wei Qi energy. Lastly, the lungs distribute liquids to the skin through the control of liquid metabolism. This is why patients suffering from asthma, bronchitis, sinus problems, and allergies usually have very dry skin. The lung's properties and characteristics are:

PROPERTY	ASPECT
Emotion	Grief, expressed vocally by weeping
Body Fluid	Mucus
Season	Autumn
Environmental Factor	Dryness
Phase of Growth	Reaping
Color	White
Taste	Pungent
Direction	West
Healing Sound	ZZZ

Lung Imbalance

Because the lung meridian extends through the intestines, the lungs, the nose and the skin, symptoms of lung imbalance can manifest in all of these areas. The most common lung imbalances are those associated with the common cold or flu. Sneezing, sinusitis, runny nose, sore throat, headache, muscle aches and pains, chills, and lack of sweat are all symptoms of lung disorders.

These symptoms are most often caused by not wearing enough clothes to protect yourself from drafts and windy days, or by sleeping without a blanket, with a window open, or with a fan blowing directly onto your body when the navel or the back of the head is exposed. The skin, the opening of the lungs, is the largest organ, and it protects us from outside invaders. When we expose it too much to the elements, it cannot sustain its protective role.

When colds and flu are not treated properly and are allowed to develop into a more acute condition, prolonged illness will result in lung Qi deficiency. The following symptoms may occur:

- excessive mucus formation

- runny nose

- thick sputum

- lack of energy, and fatigue,

- a tendency to sweat with very little exertion

- shortness of breath

The health of the lungs will be affected by other organ systems as well, and vice versa. The breath inhaled through the nose and lungs is dependent on the ability of the kidney energy to refine it. Therefore, a lung Qi problem will affect the kidney. For example, a person experiencing a kidney deficiency will usually have allergies and sinus problems. Likewise, a prolonged lung problem will weaken the kidney energy. The connection between the two can often be observed in people with low back pain. If they sneeze and feel discomfort in the area of the back where their back pain is evident, it is indicative of a lung Qi deficiency that has affected the kidney.

Weakened health or a problem in the colon may also manifest symptoms in the lung system. A blocked bowel movement is often accompanied by a sinus problem. People often attribute sneezing and sinusitis with an allergic reaction, but it may actually be caused by too many toxic substances in the large intestine. The nose serves as a flue to help rid the internal organs of poisonous toxins; if the toxins become excessive, the body can develop sinus conditions. The pores of the skin and body hair are also affected in this elimination chain.

Lastly, when someone experiences grief, the emotion associated with the lungs, they often experience coughing or chest pain and the skin will feel excessively wet or dry. Since the lungs are also closely related to the colon, this grief can cause constipation or diarrhea.

Dreams

When the energy of the lungs is exhausted, one dreams of white objects or the cruel killing of people. If there is excessive lung energy, one dreams of being frightened or of crying. In cases of extreme deficiency of lung energy, one dreams of soaring through the air or seeing strange objects made of metal.

Seasonal Sickness

Changes in the weather can lead to a lung imbalance or seasonal sicknesses commonly known as colds or flu. Take the following precautions to protect yourself:

1. If you are used to sleeping in clothes, wear light cotton pajamas and cover the abdomen with a cotton towel to protect the "sea of Qi" from the entry of negative energy during sleep.

(The area approximately 1½ inches below the umbilicus is known as the "sea of Qi" because it is where energy from various sources collects to be channeled throughout the body.)

2. Wear adequate clothing on a day that is cloudy, windy, rainy, or dark. Remember, clothing is worn to protect yourself. An important thing to consider is that we are a small microcosmic universe within the largest macrocosmic universe. When it is dark, cloudy, windy, or stormy outside, our bodies may experience similar symptoms inside. By wearing adequate clothing you will lessen the work that the skin and lung organ has to do to perform its protective role.

Massage

A massage is often helpful in restoring lung balance when you have a cold or flu. It should be executed without oils because they will block the pores which will then be prevented from eliminating toxins out of the circulatory system. After a massage, drink warm ginger tea, go to bed, and cover yourself with a blanket to promote perspiration.

KIDNEYS

The kidneys are located on either side of the lumbus. They are energetically associated with the reproductive organs and functions. The kidney meridian is related to the urinary bladder and opens out to the ears.

The main physiological functions of the kidneys are the storage of the life essence and the domination of reproduction, growth, and development. The essence of the kidneys (also referred to as the "yin" of the kidneys) consists of two parts: (1) congenital essence inherited from the parents and (2) acquired essence transformed from the essential substances in food.

Just as the moon continually receives the light of the sun, the kidneys are continually receiving and storing the essence of life that originates from the universe. The kidneys, in turn, transmute this energy into Qi. The kidney is also the recipient of the Qi that has been transmuted by the lungs. The processing of the pure Qi inhaled by the lungs and distributed throughout the body is not only dependent on the descending function of the lungs but also on the ability of the kidneys to receive and refine it. This, in turn, is regulated by the spleen.

The *Nei Ching* gives precise descriptions of the physiological function of the kidney Qi in the 4-phase process of birth, growth, full development, and senility. The kidney Qi begins to flourish at about age of 14 in women and 16 in men. (It may be a little earlier in America.) Women experience the onset of menstruation, and men develop seminal emission, both signifying the power of reproduction. The Qi of the kidney is highest at the age of 28 in women and about 32 in men, when the body is fully developed and in its prime. When women reach the age of 49 and men are about 64, the Qi of the kidneys starts to decline, the body begins to wither, and the function of reproduction gradually fails. This process unfolds painlessly if one takes care of oneself through proper food consumption, maintaining emotional balance, and making sure environmental conditions enhance the quality of life. Each factor can make a significant contribution for better or worse.

The kidney Qi also plays a significant role in the production of marrow, the formation of brain tissue, the domination of the bones, and the manufacture of blood. The condition of the kidney Qi in these functions can be determined by examining the hair on the head, which is an outward manifestation of its energy.

Another important function of the kidney is the domination of water metabolism. The kidney is the recipient of the fluid that descends from the activity of the lungs. The yang function of the kidney divides it into two parts: clear and turbid. The clear fluid, which contains useful nutrients, is retained; the turbid fluid flows into the urinary bladder to be excreted as urine.

The connection of the kidney meridian to the ears is interesting and warrants some explanation. The ears reflect the kidneys in their shape and form. Just as the tongue, the opening of the heart meridian, mirrors the heart, so the ears indicate the essence of the kidneys. A crescent moon shape would indicate something different than an oblong shape. Since the ears cannot physically be closed (unlike the eyes or mouth), they are always open and always receiving. Likewise, the kidneys are always open and receiving and processing the vital energy essence. Because of this connection to the ears, deafness in aged people is mainly due to a deficiency in the Qi of the kidney. Following are the properties and aspects of the kidneys:

PROPERTY	ASPECT
Emotion	Fear, vocally expressed by groaning
Body Fluid	Urine
Season	Winter
Environmental factor	Cold
Phase of growth	Storing
Color	Gray, deep blue, brown, or black
Taste	Salty
Direction	North
Healing sound	CHWAY

Kidney Imbalance

We are living in a very stressful society, which requires energy to meet demands that come from many directions—jobs, relationships, financial concerns, and pollution, just to mention a few. There is the stress of wondering if you will develop a major illness which in itself could be caused by stress.

In my native country, when you say you will meet someone at noon tomorrow at their office, it means sometime around noon. Here, noon means 12 o'clock; if you arrive five minutes after 12, you are late. So it can be stressful just to think about being on time for your appointments. Finally, there is the stress of overcoming stress. All of this is traumatic to the nervous system.

Stress is closely or directly related to fear. Fear will eventually deplete the kidney energy. In addition, consuming too many foods that drain the kidney yang and engaging in excessive sexual activity will impair or weaken the function of the kidney. The foods that debilitate kidney Qi and the resulting symptoms which might manifest are outlined below.

FOODS WHICH DEPLETE KIDNEY QI	SYMPTOMS OF KIDNEY QI DEPLETION
sugar	low back pain
alcohol	knee pain
coffee	chronic fear, anxiety, worry
chocolate	lack of motivation and self-confidence
beer	forgetfulness
citrus juices	ringing in the ears
black tea	loss of head hair
	infertility
	hearing loss

[PLEASE NOTE: foods in this table are not directly related to the symptoms across from them.]

The liver Qi has an important connection and influence upon the healthful functioning of the kidney Qi; this relationship should be clearly understood when trying to determine the source of imbalances. The liver (wood element) depends on the kidney (water element) to moisten and nurture it. Water is the mother of wood. When stress weakens the kidney energy, the liver Qi rebels, causing symptoms of anger and frustration. This will cause the liver energy to rise. When the liver energy rises toward the upper part of the body, rather than descending as it should under balanced conditions, it will cause the lung energy and fluid from the middle burner to ascend. This combination of rebellious Qi and fluid toxins may manifest in a number of primary and underlying symptoms and emotions, as shown below.

PRIMARY SYMPTOMS	UNDERLYING SYMPTOMS	UNDERLYING EMOTIONS
allergic rhinitis	fatigue	fear, anxiety, worry
watery eyes	reduced sex drive	loudness
sinus headache	cold feet	anger
excess mucus in the chest	low back, neck, and shoulder pain	frustration, confusion
hives	susceptibility to cold and flu	impatience
	sciatica	premature ejaculation
	neuralgia	uneasiness
	arthralgia	"heavy spirit"
	impulsive eating due to nervousness	too much sensory awareness thinking of negative thoughts

Dreams

When the energy of the kidney is exhausted, one may dream of a ship full of drowning men or of lying in water and becoming frightened. In extreme cases of kidney energy depletion, one dreams of approaching a ravine and plunging into water. When the kidney energy is in excess, one dreams of a sensation that the back and waist can no longer be stretched and are split apart.

GALL BLADDER

The gall bladder is attached to the liver. Its main functions are to store bile and aid in excretion. In this way it assists the intestine in its digestive functions and also helps the liver to increase the potency of its vital energy. It participates in the assimilation of food but not in its ingestion and transformation.

The gall bladder influences the circulation of the nourishing (Yin) and protective (Wei) energies of the body. While the liver has the ability to plan, the gall bladder has the ability to decide. For this reason, it is titled the "Minister of Justice" of the body. Only when the liver and gall bladder are equally healthy will an individual demonstrate courage and decisiveness.

Dreams

According to the *Nei Ching*, a deficiency in gall bladder energy will cause one to dream of engaging in flight and battles, or of cutting open one's own body.

SMALL INTESTINE

The small intestine is situated in the abdomen. Its upper end is connected to the stomach by the pylorus. Its main function is to receive and temporarily store partially digested food, to separate coarse substances from the fine, and to absorb nourishing substances, along with some water.

Dreams

Extreme deficiencies of small intestine energy will cause one to dream of populous town districts and main thoroughfares.

STOMACH

The stomach is situated in the epigastrium. Its upper outlet is connected by the cardia to the esophagus, and its lower outlet communicates with the small intestine by way of the pylorus. Its main function is to receive and decompose food. It is referred to as the "sea of nourishment." It functions in relationship with the spleen.

The *Nei Ching* describes the stomach: "The stomach is the sea of the internal organs. Since food comes to the organs via the stomach, the stomach is their sea of energy." The stomach governs digestion; it sends the essence from food to the spleen for circulation and distribution. The stomach and spleen together are often referred to as the source of health.

Dreams

A deficiency of stomach energy will cause one to dream of eating or drinking.

LARGE INTESTINE (COLON)

The large intestine is situated in the abdomen. Its upper end is connected to the small intestine by the ileocecum, and its lower end exits to the exterior of the body through the anus. The main function of the large intestine is to receive the waste materials sent down from the small intestine. It functions as a conduit in which the assimilation and temporary storage of food takes place. As waste materials are being transported to the anus, the large intestine absorbs a part of the fluid and turns the remainder into fecal matter to be excreted.

Dreams

A deficiency in the energy of the large intestine will cause dreams of fields and rural landscapes.

URINARY BLADDER

The urinary bladder is situated in the lower abdomen. It is related to the kidney, and its main functions are the temporary storage of urine and the discharge of urine from the body when a certain amount has been accumulated. The function of the urinary bladder is assisted by the Qi from the kidney.

The *Nei Ching* describes the bladder as the "provincial officer in charge of liquid." The excess fluids of the body converge and are stored in the urinary bladder. Some excess fluid evaporates as sweat, and some passes out with fecal matter, but most of it descends to the urinary bladder for evacuation.

Dreams

A deficiency in the energy of the urinary bladder will cause one to dream of talking, walking, and taking an excursion.

BRAIN

In Chinese medicine the brain is in the category of extraordinary organs. Its functions are dominated by various organs, with the heart having the main influence. The heart houses the energy which feeds the mind, and the liver regulates the functioning of the nervous system and the potency of vital functions. Thus, both organs are intimately related to the brain's mental activities.

The *Nei Ching* describes the brain as a "sea of marrow." As mentioned earlier, the kidney produces the marrow that forms the brain. The filling of the "sea," then, is dependent on the essence of the kidney. A healthy and steady mind, then, is greatly dependent upon the health of the heart, liver, and kidney energy systems.

UTERUS

The function of the uterus is to preside over menstruation and nourish the fetus. It is related to the kidneys. Only if the kidney energy is sufficient can the menstrual cycle occur regularly and impregnation and growth of the fetus take place. Like the brain, the uterus is in the category of extraordinary organs in Chinese medicine.

TRIPLE BURNER

The triple burner is a concept unfamiliar to Western medicine. It is not a physical organ but rather a method of dividing the main body into three groups of physiological functions.

As shown in the triple burner diagram, the three groups of physiological functions are:

1. Upper Burner (representing the chest)—encompasses the functions of the heart and lungs in transporting the Qi and blood to nourish various parts of the body.

2. Middle Burner (representing the epigastrium)—encompasses the functions of the spleen and stomach in assisting digestion and absorption. The middle burner is of particular importance because it is the foundation of postnatal life and the source of acquired essence.

3. Lower Burner (representing the hypogastrium)—encompasses the functions of the kidneys, liver, large and small

intestines, and urinary bladder in controlling water metabolism, as well as storage and excretion of urine. This is the pathway for the flow of water throughout the body.

The energy of the triple burner extends through the membranes of the body cavity. The membranes and fat deposits provide protection for the organs and regulate body temperature. The triple burner influences the supply of blood, Qi, and fluids to the muscles, skin, and other organs.

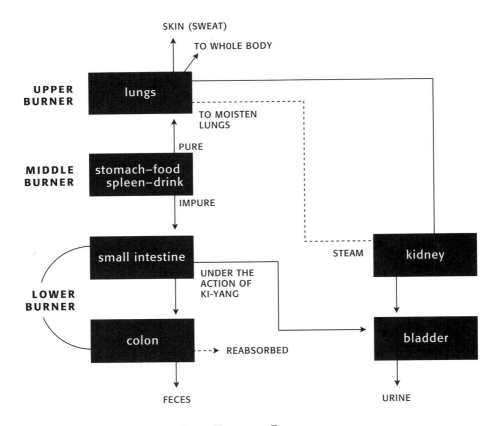

THE TRIPLE BURNER

As the mechanism for transformation of the essence energy, it is also the source of protective energy or Wei Qi.

The balanced flow of energy throughout the organs of the triple burner facilitates the functioning of the pericardium in maintaining the order of energy to the heart. This nourishment energy (ying) is the essence that fires the kundalini experience, wherein the eternal oneness of the God force is experienced. For this reason, traditional Chinese medicine considers the triple burner as a functioning unit to be as important in diagnosis as all other body systems.

Triple Burner Imbalance

A high fever, which accompanies some diseases, is often the result of the malfunction of the triple burner and associated membranes. If the membranes become constricted, energy flow is impeded and heat builds inside the trunk of the body. On the other hand, when the membranes are too loose, energy will leak out unchanneled, reducing vitality and making one tire easily. All the organs that make up the triple burner need the warm embrace of resilient membranes to maintain good energy flow.

An impairment of the middle burner is the cause of stomach disorders. When the middle burner is impaired, the body cannot extract the pure Qi from food. The following symptoms may be evident:

- indigestion

- poor appetite

- abdominal distention

- fatigue

- tendency toward loose stool

- chronic diarrhea

- gastric or duodenal ulcers

- anemia

- a pale tongue with thin fur

The nature of the spleen is dryness, and the stomach nature is dampness, so if the spleen is too damp, there will be an obstruction of the upward flow of spleen energy. If the problem is not corrected, there will be a drain on the root energy of the middle burner, leading to a deficiency of yang energy. An advanced case of yang deficiency will exhibit further symptoms:

- fear of cold and a desire for warmth

- a desire for hot food and drink

- cold hands and cold feet

- watery stool, possibly containing undigested food

- the tongue will be moist, pale, and swollen, with teeth prints on both sides.

FIVE LEVELS OF PURIFICATION

This section will tie together all the concepts that have been presented thus far. It will show how the Yin/Yang Theory, The Law of the Five Elements, and the function of the organs are all related to the maintenance of strong Qi and how they interact in refining energy for the body. Most importantly, this section will explain the vital role food plays in protecting the body from outside invasion.

The forces of yin and yang are present from the outset. The earth (yin energy) provides the food that enters the stomach (yang organ).

Heaven (yang energy) provides the air for breath that enters the lungs (yin organ). Movement is caused by the interaction of these yin and yang forces both in the environment and within the body. (Please refer to the diagram showing the five levels of purification.)

Stimulated by the physical laws of attraction and repulsion characteristic of the yin/yang dynamic, digested food in liquid form moves from the stomach (yang, hollow organ) to the spleen (yin, solid organ) to be transformed into the essence energy that will be distributed to the other organs for absorption. The same dynamic of attraction and repulsion occurs between all pairs of hollow and solid organs as they work together to stimulate body processes. If you have been eating properly and your system is functioning well, the spleen will work in conjunction with the gastric juices in the pylorus of the stomach to produce the energy that is necessary to initiate the process of The Five Levels of Purification.

THE FIRST LEVEL OF PURIFICATION

After digested food has been transformed by the spleen, it is sent to the small intestine. Here, the energy is broken down into two parts: the pure essence travels to the kidneys along the pathway of the internal channel (not to be confused with the channels of the primary meridians discussed earlier), and combines to form Zong Qi, previously defined as the combination of the essence energy of food and Acquired Qi; the impure essence settles in the colon (large intestine).

THE SECOND LEVEL OF PURIFICATION

The Second Level of Purification occurs in the colon where the essence received is again broken down into two parts, with the pure essence serving to moisten the mucus of the colon and the impure essence traveling to the anus as feces.

THE THIRD LEVEL OF PURIFICATION

The Third Level of Purification occurs in the kidney. The separation process that occurs here sends pure essence to the liver. This is in accordance with the Law of the Five Elements, whereby water (represented by the kidney) produces wood (represented by the liver). Or, stated another way, "the kidney is the mother of the liver." The impure essence from this separation is sent to the urinary bladder.

THE FOURTH LEVEL OF PURIFICATION

The urinary bladder is the location of the Fourth Level of Purification. The impure essence that results from the separation process is excreted from the body in the form of urine, and the pure essence moves to the gall bladder.

THE FIFTH LEVEL OF PURIFICATION

Through the interaction of yin/yang forces, the essence of the gall bladder unites with that of the liver at the Fifth Level of Purification. The impure liquid from the liver is green. This green liquid travels to the gall bladder and mixes with the pure liquid from the urinary bladder to form bile, which also becomes green. This is stored in the gall bladder and drawn upon by the pylorus of the stomach as needed, to aid in the digestive process.

As stated earlier, the liver is the site of the actual formation of Wei Qi energy. The pure essence created at the Fifth Level of Purification concentrates in the liver while we sleep and is eventually transformed into steam. Following the rotation cycle of the organs, the peak time for the liver is between 1:00 AM and 3:00 AM (Please see the table following). By the time we are ready to wake, the cycle of the Five Levels of Purification is complete and Wei Chi energy is ready to go to work.

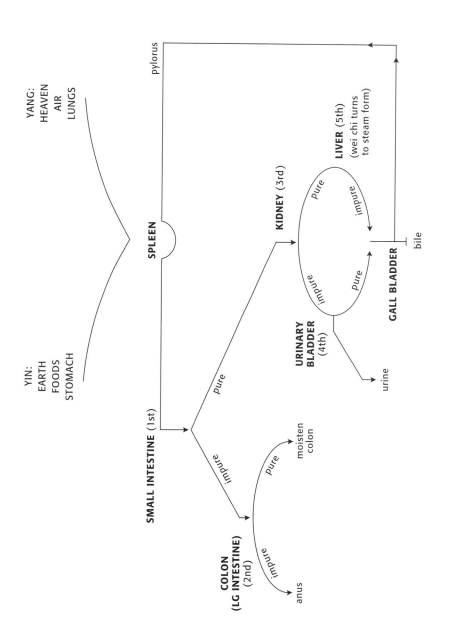

YANG:
HEAVEN
AIR
LUNGS

YIN:
EARTH
FOODS
STOMACH

pylorus

SPLEEN

KIDNEY (3rd)

LIVER (5th)
(wei chi turns
to steam form)

pure

impure

GALL BLADDER

bile

**URINARY
BLADDER**
(4th)

impure

pure

urine

SMALL INTESTINE (1st)

pure

impure

moisten
colon

pure

**COLON
(LG INTESTINE)**
(2nd)

impure

anus

THE FIVE LEVELS OF PURIFICATION

THE TIME CLOCK

Our bodies are constantly responding to a biological time clock that causes the generating energies of each organ to activate on a rotational continuum. This is a daily cycle of energy that corresponds to the earth's complete rotation within a 24-hour time period. The cycle rotates through a different organ every two hours during which time that organ is functioning at its peak energy.

The pathway of this rotational continuum starts at the lungs and ends with the liver, where Wei Qi energy is formed. This pathway is governed by the Law of the Five Elements, whereby each organ both receives energy that it will utilize from the organ preceding ("the mother") and produces the energy that will be utilized by the organ following ("the son").

Eating regular meals is important for the most efficient functioning of the organs in completing the process of the Five Levels of Purification. This will ensure that the system will not be overloaded, and it will take advantage of the peak functioning times. Ignoring these natural laws will only lead to system imbalances.

By keeping the following table in mind, you can stay attuned to the natural rhythms of your organs. With an awareness of this continuum, you will be able to work more effectively toward enhancing the well-being of your entire system.

PEAK TIME PERIOD FOR EACH ORGAN

3:00 AM - 5:00 AM	Lungs
5:00 AM - 7:00 AM	Colon
7:00 AM - 9:00 AM	Stomach
9:00 AM - 11:00 AM	Spleen
11:00 AM - 1:00 PM	Heart
1:00 PM - 3:00 PM	Small Intestine

3:00 PM - 5:00 PM	Urinary Bladder
5:00 PM - 7:00 PM	Kidneys
7:00 PM - 9:00 PM	Pericardium
9:00 PM - 11:00 PM	Triple Burner
11:00 PM - 1:00 AM	Gall Bladder
1:00 AM - 3:00 AM	Liver

THE INFLUENCE OF THE SEASONS

Just as we experience a daily cycle of change, the annual seasonal progression has a significant effect on our bodies. As the earth rotates, all of its living forms experience changes in their patterns of growth and development, and humans are no exception. We can enhance our well-being by being aware of these changes and making appropriate adjustments to our daily routines. To flow with the peak energies of this natural seasonal cycle is part of the simple path. The four seasons are briefly described below, along with helpful suggestions which can greatly influence the maintenance of your health.

SPRING/LIVER ENERGY

Spring is the time for all living things to begin to germinate and grow. It is a time for cleaning house and shaping things up for the summer. So it is with the body. One should go to bed early at nightfall and get up early at sunrise.

SUMMER/HEART ENERGY

Summer is the time when the energy from the sky pours downward and the energy from the earth rises. One should go to bed late and get up early. Avoid getting angry early in the morning, and keep the spirit lively and pleasant.

AUTUMN / LUNG ENERGY

Autumn is the time when all things are ripe and ready to harvest. The weather is cool, and plants look solitary. One should go to bed early and get up in the morning at daylight. Emotions should be calm and peaceful and lung energy should be purified.

WINTER / KIDNEY ENERGY

Winter is the time when all living things withdraw and conserve. Nature shows an overall condition of hidden yang energy. One should go to bed early and get up only when the sun is in the sky. As when we are truly contented, emotions should not be allowed to be too explicit, and we should avoid activities that allow too much energy to escape through sweating.

food as energy

Eastern Principles of Nutrition

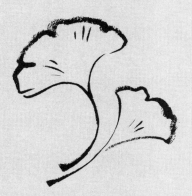

PLEASE NOTE: While garlic and onion are mentioned in the discussion of food in this book and are included in some of the later recipes, I would like to caution readers to use these foods in moderation. Feel free to omit garlic and/or onion entirely from any recipe or from your diet.

THE NATURE
AND ACTION OF FOOD

*i*n Western medicine, foods are understood by their chemical components and structure. Nutritional charts give information on the amounts of proteins, carbohydrates, fats, and vitamins. This information is primarily focused on using food in weight loss diets. There is little understanding, however, on how different foods interact with the body's energy system and how food can be used to promote the vitality of the body. In Chinese medicine, food is considered for its energetic qualities and actions. It is understood that food contains within it a vital energy essence which is used in the maintenance and development of the body's own energy. Different foods, with different energetic qualities, will have different effects upon the system. Thus by understanding the nature of foods, Chinese medicine uses foods and herbs in treating most human ailments.

In the oriental system, foods have three main properties or qualities: The Five Natures or Energies, the Four Movements, and the Five Flavors. The Five Natures refer to the heat energy of food and its potential to generate heating or cooling effects in the human body. This does not only have to do with the temperature of the food in preparation but with its innate energetic quality. The Four Movements relates to the understanding that foods, when transmuted into energy, have four distinct directions within the body to which they will naturally disperse. The Five Flavors categorize foods by their taste quality. The tastes are each related to the Five Elements and affect the organs associated with that element.

In treating illness, the oriental practitioner prescribes food with the energetic qualities to stimulate or check an energy pattern in the body and bring the system gently back into harmony. For example, if a person is exhibiting a "cold" illness, such as a cold or flu, they will tend to need "hot" or "warm" foods. If they are exhibiting symptoms of an upward moving disorder, such as vomiting or hiccuping, they will benefit from downward moving foods, such as bananas or mangoes. If a person needs to stimulate circulation, bitter foods which corresponds to the fire element and the heart would be prescribed. A thorough understanding of illnesses, the nature of foods, and the basic constitution of the individual is necessary to predict the effect of foods on the metabolism and physiology of a person's body.

THE FIVE NATURES

The Five Natures or Energies of food are hot, warm, neutral, cool, and cold. These refer to the effect of food on the metabolism and physiology of the human body. Hot foods (such as ginger and cayenne pepper) create more warmth for the body and stimulate circulation. Cold foods (such as bananas and mung beans) have a cooling effect.

The *Nei Ching* expresses Chinese medical heteropathy when it says, "If it is cold, heat it; if it is hot, cool it." Therefore, warm or hot food is used to treat a cold or cool disease. For example, pepper, ginger and alcohol are "hot" foods. They tend to generate heat in the body. Lettuce, grapefruit, and watermelon are cold foods, which will cool the body down. The following is a categorization of a few foods by their natures:

THE NATURES OF SELECTED FOODS

Hot Foods	Warm Foods	Neutral Foods	Cool Foods	Cold Foods
Alcohol	Brown sugar	Adzuki beans	Apples	Bamboo shoots
Cinnamon bark	Chives	Apricots	Barley	Bananas
Dried ginger	Cinnamon twig	Beef	Chicken	Chestnuts
Fried foods	Cloves	Carrots	Cucumbers	Crab
Greasy foods	Coffee	Celery	Mangoes	Grapefruit
Pepper	Egg yolk	Chinese cabbage	Mung beans	Ice cream
Rich foods	Fresh ginger	Duck	Pears	Kelp
Spices (most)	Ginseng	Egg white	Radishes	Lettuce
	Grapefruit peel	Figs	Sesame seeds	Oranges
	Ham	Grapes	Strawberries	Salt
	Leeks	Honey	Tangerines	Seagrass
	Mutton	Kidney beans	Turnips	Seaweed
	Nutmeg	Milk (cow, human)	Wheat	Soft drinks
	Peaches	Olives		Sorbet
	Raspberries	Oysters		Sour foods
	Rosemary	Peanuts		Water chestnuts
	Shrimp	Pineapples		Watermelon
	Sunflower seeds	Plums		
	Sweet basil	Polished rice		
	Walnuts	Pork		
	Wine	Potatoes		
		Pumpkin		
		Radish leaves		
		Rice (whole grain and sweet)		
		Sweet potatoes		

THE FOUR MOVEMENTS

According to Chinese medicine food that has been transmuted into energy moves to four distinct areas when digested. These are:

1. the inside or internal organs

2. the outside or skin surface

3. the upper body, or waist and above

4. the lower body, or below the waist.

The movements corresponding to these areas are:

- Inward or Sinking Movement

  Foods that tend to move toward the center and affect the inner parts of the body. They will promote the function of the bowels and clear up swelling in the abdomen.

- Outward or Floating Movement

  Foods that tend to stay toward the surface of the body or near the skin. They will help reduce fever by inducing perspiration.

- Upward or Ascending Movement

  Foods which affect the upper body regions rather than the lower areas. Eating upward-moving foods will reduce, balance, or reverse illnesses that have a downward motion such as diarrhea and prolapse.

- Downward or Descending Movement

  Foods that move downward from the upper body to the lower body. Such foods will relieve the effects of upward afflictions like vomiting, hiccups, asthma, and coughing.

THE MOVEMENT OF SELECTED FOODS

Inward Movement	Outward Movement	Upward Movement	Downward Movement
Crab	Black pepper	Apricots	Apples
Hops	Cinnamon bark	Beef	Bamboo shoots
Kelp	Dried ginger	Beet root	Bananas
Lettuce	Green pepper	Black sesame seeds	Barley
Salt	Red pepper	Chinese cabbage	Bean curd
Seaweed	Soybean oil	Carrots	Chicken egg white
	White pepper	Celery	Cucumbers
		Chicken egg yolk	Eggplant
		Duck	Grapefruit
		Grapes	Lettuce
		Honey	Litchi nuts
		Kidney beans	Loquats
		Milk	Mangoes
		Olives	Mung beans
		Oysters	Mushrooms
		Peanuts	Peaches
		Pork	Persimmons
			Spinach
			Strawberries
			Sugarcane
			Tangerines
			Water chestnuts
			Watermelon

THE FIVE FLAVORS

According to the *Nei Ching*, each element creates a particular flavor which enters, strengthens, and nourishes a particular organ and is proper food for that particular organ. In learning to promote your own well-being through food, it is important to understand how the five flavors enter each organ and how the flavors can be balanced for healing and enhancing health.

Each flavor has a special power, influence, or effect on another flavor and organ. The *Su Wen*, an important oriental medicine text, speaks of the "Travels of the Five Flavors" in the following quote: "Sour travels to the liver. Pungent travels to the lungs. Bitter travels to the heart. Salt travels to the kidney. Sweet travels to the spleen. And these are called the five entering routes." The *Ling Shu* delineates the ultimate destination of the five flavors in this quote: "Each of the five tastes moves to what it likes. Sour travels to the tendons. Pungent travels to the Qi. Bitter travels to the blood. Salt travels to the bones. Sweet travels to the flesh. Such are called the five travels."

THE FIVE ELEMENTS AND THE TRAVELS OF THE FIVE FLAVORS

Element:	Creates the Flavor:	Power of Flavor Is:	Flavor Travels To:	Flavor's Final Destination:
Wood	Sour	Astringent / gathering	Liver	Tendons
Fire	Bitter	Drying / strengthening	Heart	Blood
Earth	Sweet	Harmonizing	Spleen	Flesh
Metal	Hot / pungent	Dispersing	Lung	Qi
Water	Salty	Softening	Kidney	Bones

Each flavor, when in excess, can be counteracted by its own special counteractor. Each can also act as a counteractor to another flavor. The table and illustration below outline the dynamics of this system.

EXCESS OF FLAVOR:	COUNTERACTS:	IS COUNTERACTED BY:
SOUR	Sweet	Pungent
BITTER	Pungent	Salty
SWEET	Salty	Sour
PUNGENT	Sour	Bitter
SALTY	Bitter	Sweet

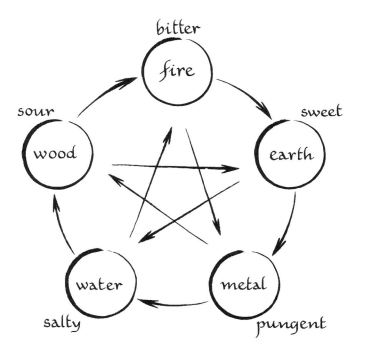

THE FIVE ELEMENTS AND THE TRAVELS OF THE FIVE FLAVORS

Following is a description of each of the five flavors, the stimulating effects they have on the organs of the body, and their relationships to the Five Elements. Notice that each flavor is directly related to two of the ten vital organs—one hollow and one solid.

BITTER

The bitter taste corresponds to the fire element and the color red. It affects the heart and small intestine and influences the bones. It clears the vessels of cholesterol, eliminates heat toxins, stimulates the circulation and digestive secretions, and removes fat and parasites. The counterbalancing taste for bitter is the pungent taste.

SWEET

The sweet taste correlates with the earth element and the color yellow. It affects the spleen and stomach and influences the flesh. It has a direct effect on the building functions of the spleen and pancreas and will help to replenish the energies of these organs. The sweet flavor has a comforting, warming, tonifying effect, which supplements deficiencies and encourages relaxation by slowing down many bodily functions. When taken in moderate amounts and in the form of balanced carbohydrates, it will help to satisfy deep cravings and desires and can neutralize the toxic effects of some foods. The sweet taste is used for its dispersing and flowing properties. The counterbalancing taste for sweetness is the salty taste.

PUNGENT

The pungent taste corresponds to the metal element and the color white. It affects the lungs and colon, and influences the Qi through a dispersing action. It induces perspiration and helps remove obstructions in the blood by promoting circulation. It can be taken to help relieve excessive fullness and generally to stimulate vitality. The counterbalancing taste for pungent is the sour taste.

SALTY

The salty taste corresponds to the water element and the colors black and dark blue. Salty flavors are used as lubricants or to disperse accumulations. Salt affects the kidneys and bladder and influences the blood by helping the body to retain the proper amount of moisture, softeners, and lubrication. It is characterized by cold energy and can impair the flow of blood and Qi by its constricting action. The bitter taste counterbalances the salty taste.

SOUR

The sour taste belongs to the wood element and the color green. Sour flavors are used for their astringent and absorbent properties. Sour affects the liver and gall bladder and influences the tendons. It also helps to stimulate the flow of internal secretions such as hormones and enzymes. The sweet taste counterbalances the sour taste.

EXCESS OF THE FIVE FLAVORS

When the diet contains an excess of one or more of the five flavors, detrimental and unbalancing effects can occur. The following outlines some of the symptoms that can result from an excess in each of the five flavors.

EXCESS SOUR

- Is injurious to the muscles
- Causes the flesh to harden, wrinkle, and become tough
- Causes the lips to become dry and slack
- Causes the liver to produce excess saliva

- Causes the force of the spleen to be cut short

- Avoid sour foods if you have arthritis and/or rheumatism.

EXCESS BITTER

- Causes the spleen energy to become dry and weakens its ability to transform and transport energy and nutrients

- Causes the stomach energy to become dense and congested

- Dries and withers the skin

- Causes the body hair to fall out

- When there is a disease of the bones, one should not eat too much bitter food.

EXCESS SWEET

- Causes aches in the bones

- Causes the heart energy to be too full, which weakens it and causes breathing difficulty

- Causes an imbalance in the kidneys, which can result in a bladder infection

- Causes the hair on the head to fall out

- May injure the flesh.

EXCESS PUNGENT

- Knots the muscles

- Slackens the muscles and pulse

- Injures the spirit, the skin, and the body hair

- Causes fingernails and toenails to wither and decay

- When there is illness of the respiratory tract, do not eat too much pungent food.

EXCESS SALTY

- Causes the great bones to become weary

- Causes a deficiency in the bones, muscles, and flesh

- Causes the mind to become despondent (in cases of depression, cut common salt out of the diet completely for a while)

- Hardens the pulse

- Causes tears to appear

- Causes the complexion to lose its vitality

- Avoid salty foods if you suffer from blood disease, a weak heart, deficiency in the spleen or kidney, or edema.

APPLYING THE LAW OF THE FIVE ELEMENTS TO FOODS

Learning to use the Law of the Five Elements will help you to know what foods are appropriate for your health, age, job situation, body condition, and the outdoor weather. Eating the right food will help assure maintenance of a healthy balance in body and mind.

There is no one best food for everyone. Diet should be tailored to each individual's needs. Some need food to detoxify, others need food to build up strength. Many need both. As we learn more about food and the therapeutic as well as energy-supplying properties it has, we will know when we need to change to different foods to keep ourselves balanced. In this way, we can fully utilize food as a resource for nourishment and healing.

As seen in the following table, each of the Five Elements has a corresponding grain, fruit, domestic animal, and vegetable that conform to each other to supply the beneficial essentials of life. In proper combination, they will assure a sound, harmonious, and healthy diet. Also listed below are the Five Elements' corresponding yin organs, yang organs, and planets.

	WOOD	FIRE	EARTH	METAL	WATER
GRAIN	Wheat	Glutinous millet	Millet	Rice	Beans or peas
FRUIT	Peach	Plum	Apricot	Chestnut	Dates
ANIMAL	Chicken or fowl	Mutton or lamb	Beef	Horse	Pig
VEGETABLE	Mallow	Coarse greens	Scallions	Onion	Leeks
YIN ORGAN	Liver	Heart	Spleen	Lung	Kidney
YANG ORGAN	Gall Bladder	Spleen	Stomach	Colon	Urinary Bladder
PLANET	Jupiter	Mars	Saturn	Venus	Mercury

FOODS TO NURTURE THE ORGANS

The five constituents of the cell are fats, electrolytes, carbohydrates, proteins, and water. Each constituent has a corresponding organ and element. A craving for any constituent probably indicates a deficiency in the respective element and a need to counterbalance the deficiency by eating foods containing the substance. This is a very simplified approach and must not be taken to an extreme. Use it as a guideline. As mentioned earlier, if you are under the care of a physician, these rules may not apply to you. The following chart will help you decide which kinds of food to eat to nurture particular organs as the dynamics of your metabolism fluctuate in response to the ever-changing matrix of your life.

ELEMENT	SUBSTANCE PROVIDED	ORGAN AFFECTED
Wood	Fat	Liver / Gall Bladder
Fire	Electrolyte	Heart / Small Intestine
Earth	Carbohydrate	Stomach / Spleen
Metal	Protein	Lungs / Colon
Water	Water	Kidney / Bladder

FOODS FOR DIFFERENT SEASONS

The Creator offers us foods each season that will address the appropriate physical, mental, and spiritual needs of our organs. By eating the foods appropriate to the season, you will stay in the flow of nature's cycle and take advantage of the peak energy of the season.

Spring / Liver Energy

We need mostly upward-moving foods to combat the effects of prolapse from the cold, physically exhausting winter. We need to combine both cool and warm foods to balance the body and prepare it for a more active summer.

Summer / Heart Energy

In the summer, it is appropriate to eat food that moves energy up and outward to the surface, that supports an increase in activity and elimination of toxins, that helps the Qi and blood circulate freely and vigorously, and that keeps the body cool. Raw tomatoes and watermelon are good to counteract summer heat. They strengthen the stomach and harmonize the liver and stomach energy.

Autumn / Lung Energy

Our bodies require the downward-moving foods, which help to compensate for the dampness that may induce nausea, vomiting, hiccups, asthma, or colds. Warming foods should be eaten when a chill is in the air.

Winter / Kidney Energy

Eat hot/warm foods characterized by inward movement. Concentrate on counteracting constricting conditions (such as constipation) caused by lack of exercise and cooler weather. This will help the circulation of fluids and enable our blood and Qi to move freely to keep us warm. It will also tonify the root (the middle burner and the kidney) and regenerate essence and repair substance.

HEALING WITH FOOD

Correcting energy imbalances which have manifested as an acute illness or in chronic symptoms in the body, mind, or spirit, starts first with understanding your particular body constitution and the origin of the imbalance. In the previous sections, we've seen an overview of how the organ systems function together and some guidelines for understanding patterns of imbalance. The information in this section will help with an understanding of your own inherent body constitution and how to use food to harmonize patterns of imbalance.

UNDERSTANDING YIN/YANG IMBALANCES

Two of the most common problems of excess and deficiency are yin/yang imbalances. A person who is overly yang or deficient in yin is a fiery person. A person who has too much yin or not enough yang is a watery person.

A fiery person contains a high degree of body heat. This overabundance of heat originates in the internal organs from excessive consumption of unhealthy foods, deficient consumption of healthy foods, or eating too many foods with hot properties and too few foods with cool properties. Fiery people display outward signs of their problems in the form of nervousness, insomnia, quick temper, and anger. These people should consume more cool, watery foods to reduce the heat.

A cool watery person is usually plump and typically cold and easily depressed—the opposite of a fiery person. Cool people need foods to increase circulation and stimulate the respiratory system, and, in general, to heat the body.

CORRECTING ORGAN IMBALANCES

Once you or your physician have determined that you have an imbalance originating from a particular organ energy system, food can be used to help restore balance to the system. The choice of food and diet will depend on the severity and nature of the imbalance. In this section I describe a number of common organ imbalances and the foods which can be used to aid in their correction.

Foods to Correct Liver Imbalances

When someone easily becomes impatient, angry, or fatigued, it is because the liver energy is depleted and needs to be restored by proper food. If you suffer from one of these symptoms, a first measure is to stop eating food that aggravates the liver, and then begin eating foods which will relax the liver directly. The following table lists the substances to avoid and the foods to eat while working to correct a liver imbalance. In addition to the foods listed, any food that nurtures the kidney yin will be of benefit, since the kidney yin is the root of the liver yin. (Please see the kidney section.)

SUBSTANCES WHICH AGGRAVATE THE LIVER	FOODS WHICH RELAX THE LIVER	
Alcohol	Beef	Kelp
Cigarette smoke	Celery	Leeks
Environmental chemicals	Chicken	Liver
Mega-doses of vitamins	Congee with mung beans	Mulberries
Sugar in any form	Crab	Mussels
Synthetic drugs	Cucumbers	Nori
	Daikon	Sesame seeds
	Ginger in soups	Turnips
	Ginger tea	Watermelon
		Veal

Foods to Correct Lung Imbalances

Common Cold or Flu

If you have developed a cold or flu, stop consuming the foods that irritate or weaken the lungs. Concentrate on foods which will promote lung balance. In addition, you should eat foods that promote the spleen and stomach energy. They are the source of the lung energy and should be fed to nourish the lungs. Shown below are foods which tend to irritate or to strengthen the lung energy, and foods which promote the stomach and spleen energy:

FOODS WHICH WEAKEN THE LUNGS	FOODS TO STRENGTHEN THE LUNGS	FOODS PROMOTING STOMACH AND SPLEEN ENERGY
Cold drinks	Congee with ginger	Almonds
Cold foods	Ginger tea with raw sugar	Apples
Eggs	Warm drinks	Artichokes
Fried foods	Warm foods	Bananas
Onions		Cantaloupe
Raw foods		Corn
		Dates
		Millet
		Papayas
		Pineapple
		Pumpkin
		Salmon
		Spinach
		Squash
		Sweet potatoes

Dry Cough

If you have a health condition where your breath is warm to hot and your throat feels dry a lot of the time causing you to cough, avoid nuts, especially peanuts, since they will irritate the esophagus and induce more dry coughing. Your diet should include foods that moisten the lungs:

- apple sauce

- barley soup

- chicken broth

- clams

- mutton

- pears

- watermelon

- yams

Lung Qi Deficiency with Thickened Sputum

If you are exhibiting signs of progressing lung Qi deficiency, such as thickened sputum, sweating, and shortness of breath, the diet should consist of herbs such as codonopsis and astragalus cooked with chicken, brown rice, or barley. Do not use honey if you have thick sputum. Other foods to include in your diet are:

- Soups: abalone soup, duck soup, nori soup, oxtail soup, tomato soup (fresh, not canned)

- Fish: fresh tuna fish, oysters

- Vegetables: carrots (not carrot juice), mushrooms, mustard greens, olives, pumpkins, squash, sweet potatoes, yams

- Rice and seeds: brown rice, sesame seeds

- Fruits: papayas, peaches, winter melon

- Other: amasake, barley malt, fresh ginger

Foods to Correct Kidney Imbalances

To help alleviate the problems associated with a kidney imbalance, foods that drain the kidney energy should be avoided, such as sugar in any form, and concentrate on foods that tonify the kidney energy, such as barley soup. The table below lists the foods that irritate the kidney energy and those that promote it.

FOODS THAT DRAIN THE KIDNEY ENERGY	FOODS THAT TONIFY THE KIDNEY ENERGY	
Alcohol	Abalone	Chicken broth
Citrus juices	Adzuki beans	Dandelion
Coffee (including decaffeinated coffee)	Amasake	Endive
Fruit juices	Apples	Lamb
Milk and milk products	Asparagus	Lotus seeds
Raw cold salads	Bananas	Melon
Sugar in any form	Barley soup	Mutton
Vitamins (in mega-doses)	Beef broth	Oysters
	Black beans	Rosemary
	Brown rice	Sweet potatoes
	Celery	Tang kuei
	Chestnuts	Tuna fish (fresh, not canned)

Foods to Correct Triple Burner and Middle Burner Imbalances

When the middle burner is impaired, the body cannot extract the pure Qi from food. Stomach disorders will manifest. Symptoms such as indigestion, gastric ulcers, chronic diarrhea, poor appetite, abdominal distention and fatigue will accompany the disorder. To help this problem, you should avoid all foods that cool the digestive fire, such as iced drinks and refrigerated foods. Food that is stale, processed, or leftover lacks fire or essence to support the stomach Qi, hence it is hard to digest. For this reason, food should be eaten within 24 hours of being cooked. This is especially important for elderly and weak people. All food should be at room temperature when cooked and eaten. Other foods to avoid when the middle burner is impaired are:

- agar

- buckwheat

- cheese

- citrus fruit

- frozen food

- fruit juice

- millet

- milk

- raw fruit

- raw salad

- salt or salty food

- seaweed

- tofu

- too much liquid with meals

- too much sugar in the form of pies, cookies, cakes, and the like

To correct a middle burner impairment, the spleen Qi needs to be tonified. Foods that promote the spleen Qi and correct spleen yang deficiency are foods that are yellow in color. Remember that the nature of the spleen/stomach is of the earth, whose associated color is yellow. The following foods are beneficial for tonifying the spleen Qi:

- Vegetables and grains: cooked squash, carrots, leeks, oats, onions, pumpkins, rutabagas, sweet potatoes, sweet rice (well-cooked), turnips, yams

- Fruits (cooked or dried): cherries, dried figs, peaches, strawberries

- Meats: anchovy, chicken, mutton, turkey

- Spices: arrowroot, black pepper, cinnamon, ginger, kudzu root, nutmeg, tapioca

- Sweeteners (in small amounts): barley malt, maple syrup, rice bran syrup

USING FOOD FLAVORS TO HARMONIZE

Each of the five flavors can also be used to help harmonize and rebalance the organ systems. Some guidelines are indicated below.

BITTER

When the spleen suffers from excess moisture, bitter foods will have a drying effect and drain the spleen of excess moisture. When the lungs suffer obstructions of the upper respiratory tract, eat bitter foods to disperse obstructions and restore the flow. In general, this taste causes purging action, tending to reduce body heat, dry up body fluids, and sometimes cause diarrhea.

SWEET

When the liver suffers from an acute attack, a condition of excessive fullness is indicated. This can be quickly counterbalanced by eating sweet foods to calm it down. A sick spleen has a tendency to work too slowly; for this condition, one should eat sweet foods to supplement and strengthen it.

PUNGENT

Since the lungs govern the skin, excess use of pungent tasting food will stimulate elimination through the pores in the form of sweat and skin excrescence. Pungent foods should be avoided when Qi is weak or liver blood is deficient because pungent's dispersing action will spread deficient energy and blood and thus further weaken the body.

Use pungent foods to drain the lungs and make them expel. When the kidneys suffer from dryness, eat pungent foods to moisten them. Pungent foods also open the pores and facilitate free circulation of saliva and fluid secretions. Eat pungent foods to supplement the liver function if it has a tendency to deteriorate.

SALTY

Eat salty foods (those seasoned with sea salt) to make the heart pliable and to strengthen it. It is said in the *Nei Ching* that the salty flavor enters into the kidneys. Salt can feed or aggravate an imbalance in the kidneys and bladder, but it can also help drain the kidneys and make them expel.

SOUR

Sour foods have an astringent or gathering effect. They cause a constricting action that is beneficial when treating diarrhea or excess perspiration, but can be detrimental to cancer, AIDS, and anemia patients by impairing Qi and blood. When the heart suffers from tardiness, indicating that it is weak, the astringent properties of sour foods can strengthen it. In connection with the liver, one uses sour food in order to drain and expel. Sick lungs have a tendency to close and bind; eat sour foods in order to make them receive (gather) what is due to them. You can also use sour foods to supplement and strengthen the lungs.

At this point, you may feel that you have read so many new facts that you will never be able to remember all of them. Don't be discouraged; your efforts are one aspect of a lifelong process of logical learning, daily application, and intuitive knowing. We are here to learn and practice what we have learned. As you integrate these new ideas into your daily life, they will grow in meaning for you. The realization you experience as you experiment with the form of your life will inspire you to go deeper into the messages you find here. Then you will be actively embracing the wisdom behind the teaching.

starting on the path

Applying the Nutrition Principles
to Daily Eating

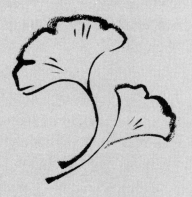

CHANGING YOUR COURSE

The first step to becoming a healthier, happier you is to decide to change. The second step it to commit to your decision. Old habits die hard, but we are never too old to change. By living a more disciplined life, you will prosper in health, emotion, and spirit. But no one will do it for you.

Keep in mind that your overall goal is a more balanced existence. With few exceptions, nothing is so bad that it will destroy you if taken in moderation, but a committed program of eating the right foods will help you achieve balance. Cooking nutritionally will not only give you the energy needed to fulfill your daily obligations but will also create the extra energy you need to go beyond these tasks to the realization of your dreams.

Be prepared to defend yourself against all of those who have not been exposed to the knowledge you have gained in your search for better health. Some may tease you about the effort you are making. Later, though, while others are still contending with persistent minor ailments (and continuing to run the risk of major problems that can stem from toxic buildup), you will be enjoying the benefits of good health, greater self-knowledge, and spiritual awakening. You will feel fortunate that your inner voice guided you onto the path that was right for you.

UNDERSTANDING THE HEALING PROCESS

In my daily practice, I am often asked an interesting question: "If my former lifestyle was so unhealthy (eating junk food, staying up late at night, drinking alcohol, smoking, etc.), why is it that I had a lot of energy; but now that I have started to take better care of myself (eating health food, getting plenty of rest, doing exercise, etc.), I sometimes get tired and don't feel well?" It is important for anyone who is going to make a successful transition to full health and vitality to know the answer to this question and have an understanding of the healing process.

When you begin a regime of eating well and exercising regularly, your body begins a process of exchanging healthy substances for unhealthy substances that have been building up in your cells for many years. When you eat junk food (coke, chocolate, candy, ice cream, alcohol, etc.), you consume large amounts of chemicals which over time become toxic to your system. They create a lot of nervous energy. You may *feel* very energetic, but this is an empty energy of hyperactivity. It has little staying power and usually leaves you feeling frayed.

These toxins and heavy energies accumulate in layers in your body over time. They prevent you from staying in touch with your inner being. This is the reason many patients tell me they don't feel "in touch" with life. Instead they feel anguish and anxiety, and they show signs of being easily intimidated by outside influences. It is only a matter of time before the empty energies carrying them through life will collapse.

As you start eating better and your body starts eliminating toxins, you will go through periods of not feeling well, then periods of feeling better, then periods not feeling well, then periods of feeling better again. This process is actually a series of body cleansings. Each time you become sick from the elimination of toxins, your body experiences what is referred to as a "healing crisis." During this time your body is throwing off an old layer of toxins and reorganizing its energy. Each time you feel better, you will notice that you feel stronger and more vital than before. Few people can make changes in their lifestyle without experiencing a certain amount of discomfort as their body chemistry and energies shift to rebalance themselves. Depending on how long and how much you have been poisoning yourself with the wrong foods you may experience this cycle to a greater or lesser degree.

Understanding this will help keep you from becoming discouraged. It is important to understand that the periods of not feeling well are actually natural and necessary parts of a healthy healing cycle. During these times, make a little extra effort to take care of yourself, conserve your energy, and nurture yourself. As time goes on, the periods of feeling well will be longer and the periods of feeling sick will be shorter, *if* you are consistent in your efforts. It took a long time for your body to build up its present level of toxicity, and it will take some time to cleanse it.

Since your body, mind, and spirit operate as one unit, ridding yourself of toxins in your physical system will help you become more aware of your center or inner being. This is the most precious part of you, the sacred part that is yours to recognize, cherish, and nourish. It guides you on a path that leads to the development of your spiritual resources. This center is very touchy and sensitive. If you mistreat your body, its temple, with unbalancing substances, energies, and stress, this center will become much more difficult to access and sustain.

As you purify your physical being, your mental and spiritual aspects open up to more pure ways of being and relating as well. You will become more aware and more sensitive to your environment. You may become more vulnerable to outside stimuli (food, negative energies, weather, environment, etc.), but this vulnerability steers you away from activities that may not be in your best interest.

For these reasons, you may at first feel worse when you are expecting to feel better as you begin to change your health habits. The important thing to remember is to be patient with yourself, and don't give up. As you become healthier, you will feel happier because you will begin to feel the calm, sustaining energies of a strong sense of inner strength and creativity. If you give up and continue to poison your body with devitalized substances, your life will eventually feel purposeless. The choice is yours.

FINDING THE TIME

A common complaint I hear when I first suggest making dietary changes to my patients is that they don't have the time. Invariably they find, however, that once they have made the transition and are in the habit, it takes them less time to prepare and cook food than before.

Initially, it will take a little time and effort buy and stock the new kinds of food you will need. This guidebook should greatly assist you in that effort. In this section I will offer you checklists of foods to stock and utensils you will need. Also, the 7-day meal plans included later in this section will make planning and shopping for the weeks quick and easy.

After the initial investment of time to stock up, I truly believe cooking time can be cut at least in half. It only takes 30 to 45 minutes a day to cook a nutritious meal. Rice will take the longest to cook—about 45 minutes depending on how much you are cooking. However, you do not have to watch over it constantly, especially if you have a rice cooker. I am convinced that once the false idea about time is surmounted, you will find more free time than you now have.

I must also mention in this regard that finding the time is mostly a matter of priorities. I have heard people say that they spend two weeks to shop for a new dress. Forty-five minutes a day toward a proper diet that will greatly enhance your quality of life and being, and will save you medical bills later, should be no great sacrifice. Our health must always be a priority, as it opens all other doors to life.

Finally, you cannot in any event achieve right consciousness without proper nutrition. All the stresses and strains and pressures created by the modern world are only exacerbated by improper eating habits. My parents used to say that no matter how modern society becomes, we should always take the time necessary to maintain the good tradition of health and well-being. I am very grateful to them for the guidance they gave me and for the opportunity to pass this wisdom on to those who are open to accepting it.

EATING WITH CONSCIOUSNESS

An old Chinese proverb says, "If a man has a happy mind, he will have a healthy body." In other words, no matter how delicious or expensive the food you eat, without a calm, relaxed, and peaceful mind, your food will not serve you as it should. In many ways, how you eat is even more important than what you eat. How you prepare and ingest food thus becomes another important way to walk the simple path.

PREPARE AND EAT IN A POSITIVE ENVIRONMENT

Like every other aspect of our phenomenal reality, food is affected by how we think about it. Therefore, the quality of food ingested is affected by the thoughts, mood, and motivation of the preparer. You can feel it when food has been prepared with love and care. Like your grandmother's cooking, it is deeply nourishing. Your system will also feel it when food has been prepared in a hurry or with disrespect.

Food should be prepared with mindfulness, respect, precision, and gratitude. When cooking, create loving energy by a positive mental attitude rather than dwelling on anything negative that might have happened to you during the day. Make an effort to get the freshest ingredients you can, clean the ingredients thoroughly, and make a beautiful presentation, even when you are just cooking for yourself.

In addition, when you eat, the atmosphere, the environment, and the feelings you receive from your surroundings are all important. In this regard, it is highly inadvisable to eat when you are nervous or upset. Under these conditions, your stomach and other organs are upset as well. Eating when you are in a hurry, in a car, or in front of the television is also detrimental to the smooth functioning of your digestive processes. Eat in a pleasant environment, free from tension and negativity. Focus on good thoughts and the act of self-nourishment.

TAKE TIME TO SAVOR AND APPRECIATE

The time you take to finish your meal is important in conscious eating. When I first came to the United States, I was invited to my sponsor's house for dinner on several occasions. At first I was embarrassed to find I was always the last one to finish my meal, and I tried to figure out why. In observing, I realized that the others were swallowing their food instead of chewing it. Later they complained of gas and indigestion. It was no wonder.

The digestion process begins in the mouth. When we chew, three glands are activated which provide saliva for digestion and send signals to the brain for timing the digestive process efficiently. This process works well when we give it enough time. By just swallowing your food, an inadequate amount of saliva will be produced and your food will not be properly neutralized before it reaches your stomach. This results in too much acidity and consequent indigestion. Additionally, when you just swallow your food, you swallow air with it, and this causes gas.

I was taught to chew each bite of food 100 times. We were told, "Drink your food and eat your drink." This means that you should chew your food thoroughly until it becomes liquid in the mouth and that you should drink liquids slowly, a little at a time, holding them in the mouth long enough for them to be mixed with saliva.

Relax and concentrate on eating your meal. Eat slowly and let your eyes "feast" on the beauty of the meal. Let your nose smell the wonderful aroma. Let your tastebuds savor every mouthful. Let your stomach become delightfully satiated. Doing so will make it easier for you to satisfy and control your hunger and appetite. You will eat less and enjoy it more.

THERE CAN BE TOO MUCH OF A GOOD THING

A good rule to follow in life as well as in proper eating habits is, "Everything in moderation. Nothing to excess." Anything taken to an extreme can be detrimental, even too much of the very food that is good for you.

I remember an incident with one of my patients that illustrates this point clearly. I told her that garlic helps reduce the thickness of blood cells, making blood clots less likely, and that it lowers serum cholesterol and triglycerides. A week later, she came in for a treatment, and I could smell her from a few feet away. I gently told her, "You may have eaten too much garlic. I can smell it from your body." She said, "Oh, no. You can never eat too much of a good food." I told her, "Yes, you can." But she persisted in her belief. A week later, she called me and was very upset. "Doctor, what should I do? My husband has terrible stomach pains." I knew immediately that it was from too much garlic. Too much of a good thing.

In this same vein, do not eat beyond the point of satiation at any one meal. A good rule of thumb is to eat only until the stomach is about 75% full. Leave some food on your plate when you feel full. Start using smaller plates to serve your food when you find yourself eating less and enjoying it more.

In short, moderation is always the best policy when learning about new foods. An excess of any activity in your daily life can damage your health. Prolonged sleep will damage energy. Prolonged sitting will damage muscles. Prolonged standing will damage bones. And prolonged walking will damage tendons. *Moderation* is the Tao way.

EAT ONLY WHEN TRULY HUNGRY

Another simple rule that may seem obvious, but which is widely disregarded, is to eat only when hungry. The pressures of our modern life cause many people to eat out of nervousness, anxiety, or boredom. They have lost touch with their natural hunger signals. Eating in this way just continually feeds energy into a pattern of agitation and stress. By eating regularly, only when you are truly hungry, you establish a regular pattern of nourishment which will generate an steady level of energy to support you throughout your day

Nervous cravings can be reduced by getting away from denatured fast foods, which do not satisfy and which create imbalances. Eating several small meals during the day rather than a few large meals might help maintain balance during times of stress and dietary transition. Drinking tea can also assist you in your efforts to maintain a good balance. Relax with a cup of freshly brewed Chinese tea to help curb an urge for something sweet. Drink it plain; it will also help cleanse the fat deposits in your gastrointestinal tract.

Do not allow the stresses and strains of your day to cause you to use food as a means of feeding your emotions or unfulfilled desires. Work on these problems by first getting in touch with their causes and then concentrating on changing them. Stresses and strains can be relieved by small efforts toward simplifying your life.

SIMPLE BALANCED NUTRITION

The following material presents the principles of oriental nutrition for maintaining balanced energy. The recommendations are necessarily general, and individuals will need to adapt them according to their specific constitutions.

THE BASIC BUILDING BLOCKS

Whole grains, legumes, vegetables, soups, meats, and fruits should be the basic building blocks of your diet. Eat these in combination with the largest portion of your diet—grains and vegetables. Keep the properties of the foods in mind when you combine them.

Raw fruit and vegetables are eliminative. Cooked grains and legumes are more building in nature. Grains and legumes are also slightly acid as a rule, while most vegetables are alkaline. Eating grains and vegetables together is an excellent way to maintain a balance between acid and alkaline foods. When you include legumes and sea vegetables you have a completely nutritious meal.

Avoid eating fruits and vegetables at the same time or at the same meal, as they are too eliminative in combination. The exceptions are avocados, pineapples, papayas, lemon juice, and lime juice, which all aid the digestive process. When protein-rich foods are eaten with other foods, eat the protein-rich foods first to allow them the most time in digestion. Refer to the section on "Basic Foods" for more detail on specific food properties.

As a general rule, the foods in your diet should be eaten according to the percentages indicated in the following categories:

PRIMARY FOODS	Whole Grains	40 – 60%
	Legumes	10%
SECONDARY FOODS	Vegetables	20 – 30%
	Soup/Seaweed	5%
OCCASIONAL FOODS	Seasonal Fruits, Meat	10 – 15%

Grains

For balanced meals, it is recommended that at least 50% of each meal be made up of whole grains such as brown rice, millet, rye, or barley. As much as possible, use organically grown whole grains.

Soup

Your meals should also be composed of 5–10% soup (1 or 2 small bowls per day). Many nutrients that are lost in cooking foods are retained in the soup broth. Eating soup will allow you to capture the full nutrients of your foods. Your soups may include grains, vegetables, and seaweed, such as wakame or kombu. Cook with miso or tamari sauce if you are a vegetarian and chicken or a beef bone if you are a meat-eater.

Vegetables

About 20–30% of each meal should consist of locally grown organic vegetables. These are extraordinary sources of minerals, enzymes, and vitamins. Most green leafy vegetables contain complete proteins of the highest quality. They should be steamed for the most part. It is fine to eat some raw salad in moderation.

Meat and Fish

If you are a meat-eater, add a small amount of white meat fish to your meals. Always make sure it is fresh. Fish that are slow moving with soft white meat (sole, founder, haddock) are yin in nature. Fish which are active with red meat (tuna, salmon, swordfish, kingfish) are yang in nature. For most people it is preferable to eat fish that are mostly yin in nature. Those who have skin allergies or dryness should avoid fish until the symptoms completely disappear.

Salads

Salads are a popular American food but do not generally promote vitality and balance in the system. They do not nourish the blood, and they cause great coldness and acid in the stomach. This is because salad is a yin food.

Yin is cold, and cold is constricting. Eating salad constricts the energy and blood flow and thus keeps food from digesting properly. Instead, the food is stored in the system as undigested material or is eventually eliminated. In either case, vital nutrients have not reached their proper destination. The body is left carrying excess baggage and is also left feeling that it needs to consume more food to be satisfied.

These are some of the factors that contribute to my clinical findings of a high incidence of low back pain, ringing in the ears, blurred vision, and low energy in general. Many obese people claim they are being calorie conscious when they restrict their lunch or dinner to a salad. I explain to them that they are perpetuating their problem by the imbalances this causes.

Salad does not require as much acid for digestion as most meats and other proteins. If you do decide to eat a salad, then the best practice is to eat high protein foods first, following them with soups and salads.

Desserts and Snacks

Dessert should be occasional and consist of fresh or dried seasonal fruit. Local and organically grown fruit is preferable. A word of caution is in order relative to eating fruit. All fruit, with the exception of melons (watermelon, cantaloupes, honeydew, etc.), have cleansing properties. This can be beneficial at times. On the whole, however, fruit should be minimized or avoided to prevent over-cleansing and depletion of energy, fluids, and vital nutrients. Women especially should not eat any fruit at all at least three days before, during, and three days after menstruation to avoid the experience of abnormal cramping and moodiness. It is best to eat fruit in moderate amounts, and it should not be eaten with any other foods.

Rice syrup and barley malt serve as acceptable sweeteners. Lightly roasted nuts are a good snack.

Beverages

As your everyday beverage, drink moderate amounts of distilled water at room temperature. Natural teas can be utilized as a substitute for coffee. They are also very nutritious and have therapeutic properties. Ginger, spearmint, peppermint, and chamomile are among the most popular. In general, though, liquids should be avoided for a period of one half hour before meals and two hours after meals.

Colors of the Five Elements

A complete and well-balanced diet is not only composed of foods offering a good variety of vitamins, minerals, and enzymes, but it should also contain a combination of complementary colors, which correspond to the Five Elements, such as:

Green from broccoli (Wood)
Yellow from yams or squash (Earth)
Red from beets or red peppers (Fire)
White from cabbage (Metal)
Black from beans (Water)

FOODS TO AVOID

There are certain foods that, due to their negative properties, disrupt the body's harmony and consequently deplete it of energy. A good general rule is to avoid foods that are processed, canned, refined, precooked, frozen, smoked, preserved, sprayed, chemically treated, or artificially colored, flavored, or sweetened. Common sense suggests that the less processing foods have undergone, the more nutrients they will have retained. No amount of "enrichment" can duplicate the wholesomeness that nature has already provided for us.

For instance, white sugar and white flour have been completely stripped of all the vital nutrients present in the original food. In the process of refinement, all vitamins, trace elements, enzymes, fatty acids, and amino acids (protein) have been removed. The final result, in the case of white sugar, is a pure crystallized form of sucrose—a pharmaceutically pure chemical. In the case of white flour, what is left is nutritionless white powder that is mostly pure starch. Eating denatured, devitalized, demineralized, and devitaminized food will inevitably lead to nutritional deficiencies.

Processed and chemically treated foods also tend to disturb the yin and yang balance of health. Since our bodies are genetically and physiologically equipped to metabolize effectively only natural whole foods, eating fragmented, refined foods will lead to metabolic disorders and biochemical imbalances. White sugar is not only an empty-calorie food, the body must draw from its own reserve supplies of vitamins and minerals just to digest it. Since our bodies are not equipped to process refined, concentrated foods, continuous ingestion of them will exert great strain on many organs and glands, eventually causing their damage and malfunction later in life.

Listed below are several categories of food that are particularly harmful. By avoiding them, you will gain a steadier, more tranquil energy and will derive greater benefit from your other health treatments.

- Iced and Cold Drinks: They shock the system and inhibit the digestive process. Remember, heat dilates and cold constricts.

- Soft Drinks/Artificial Drinks: The synthetic processing, sugar, and preservatives slowly contaminate and degenerate your system.

- Coffee (decaffeinated and regular), Colored Tea, and all Aromatic Stimulant Teas: All are strong stimulants and contain a number of toxins that cause degenerative problems.

- Alcohol, Cigarettes, Drugs: Alcohol causes extreme liver heat, which is evidenced by redness of the eyes and face. Cigarettes are obviously very harmful to the lungs. Drugs exacerbate all system imbalances.

- White Sugar and White Flour: These foods are overly refined and will lead to metabolic disorders and biochemical imbalances.

- Milk and Dairy Products: Eggs, cheese, ice cream, and milk cause mucus to form and accumulate in the body. When combined with toxins, these accumulations cause cysts and ultimately tumors.

- Juices: Processing and high acidity cause digestive problems.

- Salads: Salad is a cold energy food that causes constriction of the blood, a contributing factor to many common ailments. It should never be eaten alone as a meal but should be combined with other foods. Also, dark green lettuce is preferable to iceberg lettuce, which is devoid of any nutritious elements.

- Red Meat/Poultry: Eating too much red meat and poultry can cause a build-up of toxins. Too much red meat also makes the blood more yin; since yin constricts, this may constrict the blood flow. A maximum amount of meat or poultry would be three ounces a day.

- Hot Spices: These increase body heat and interfere with digestive processes. Use them in moderation and preferably in the fall and winter. Cut down in the summer and spring.

DRINKING LIQUIDS

The average American diet consists of too many foods that create excess body heat, such as french fries, soft drinks, hot dogs, ham, etc. Many western nutritionists recommend drinking eight glasses of water a day, which may help diminish the degenerative effects of excess heat. However, eating a wholesome balanced diet will eliminate the need for so much water.

Drinking liquids during a meal also contributes to poor health. It dilutes the necessary stomach acid needed for efficient digestion. The body, then, through its sensing mechanisms, strains itself to adjust to this diluted condition by producing more digestive acid in trying to reestablish the proper concentration. After thirty or forty years of overtaxing itself this way, its capacity to produce even the proper amount of acid has been greatly diminished and it is left needing the outside assistance of digestive aids.

Excess liquid intake also expands the stomach, reducing the elasticity of its muscle tone and thus decreasing its effectiveness in digestion. This tends to increase appetite by decreasing the satisfaction received from the food you eat. It also upsets the communication between the stomach and the spleen. This is important because, as stated previously, the spleen's function is to accept the essence of digested food from the stomach and distribute it to the rest of the body for nourishment.

Kidney deficiencies are also reliable indicators of excess liquid intake, since the kidneys dominate water metabolism. These deficiencies include excessive urination, bags under the eyes, hair falling out, knee pain, back pain, and too much self-doubt or fear. All these imbalances can be avoided by learning to eat meals without "washing down" your food.

Juices

Millions of Americans get up every morning and drink a glass of orange juice with a piece of toast. When you drink eight ounces of orange juice, you are ingesting the equivalent of seven to eight oranges. If you were eating whole oranges, you would be full by the second or third. Your system was not designed to process juice in this form and quantity efficiently. The very important action of the saliva gland is totally bypassed when juice is consumed in this way. The balancing substances in the pulp are also completely discarded.

Take carrot juice, for example. It is loaded with sodium nitrates and nitrites, which are liberated from the cellulose when juiced by a high-powered pulp-extracting juicer. This is a substance you would not digest if you ate the whole carrot. Normally, your body cannot digest cellulose in its unjuiced form and therefore passes it through the digestive system in the form of roughage with the sodium nitrate properly contained within it.

Water

Water is a basic and important factor in cooking. Because of the risk of ingesting toxic chemicals in tap water, it is always safest to have it tested by an expert or to use a water purifier.

Even bottled water cannot always be trusted. A *New York Times* reporter estimated that three-fourths of the bottled water sold in this country is not natural mineral water but rather processed water from local taps. Check with the producer when in doubt. Distilled water can be trusted to be pure as long as it has, in fact, been distilled.

Your body contains a great deal of water which it continually needs replenished. You cannot depend on coffee, tea, alcohol, or soft drinks to do this. They are all diuretics and will eventually cause an upset in your fluid balance, as they eliminate water from your system. The best drink is always pure water.

NUTRITIOUS PREPARATION

Timing Meals

Everyone should eat three good meals a day, but it is especially important to have a good breakfast between 7:00 and 9:00 in the morning. This is the peak time for the stomach and is when the stomach has the most gastric acid to aid digestion. It is advisable to have a good carbohydrate breakfast, rather than one that emphasizes protein, to give the body energy to operate for the day. Conversely, dinner should be eaten at least three hours before sleeping to allow your stomach time to settle. If absolutely necessary to eat closer to bedtime, eat some seaweed soup.

Try to allow approximately four hours between meals. This will help your stomach efficiently complete its job of digesting food and eliminating waste. Try to set and stick to definite mealtimes, within reasonable limits. In this way, your body can regulate to the times you eat, making your digestive processes most efficient and keeping your energy levels more steady.

Food Temperature

Cold food and drinks shock the nervous system and constrict the flow of blood to the brain. That is why when you drink ice water, you feel a numbness in your forehead. Cold foods have a strong effect in inhibiting circulation. I also find a strong connection between the ingestion of cold drinks and food with premenstrual syndrome in women and nervousness in men. I recommend eating food and drink at body temperature.

Cooked or Raw

Most experts recommend eating as many foods as possible in their raw state because cooking can substantially destroy the food's nutritional values. Proteins and fats, for example, become less assimilable when damaged by heat. There are, however, some important exceptions to this recommendation. Some plants contain substances, such as oxalic acid, which can be harmful when consumed in large quantities. Spinach, broccoli, asparagus, cauliflower, and vegetables in the cabbage family fall into this category.

Many vegetables can be eaten raw in the form of green salad. Others, such as potatoes, yams, squash, green beans, and those mentioned above should be lightly steamed, baked, or boiled.

VITAMINS, MINERALS, AND ENZYMES

Vitamins

The stressful society in which we live makes it difficult to get enough nourishment from food. Many people depend on vitamins to make up for the deficiencies in our diet. This practice, however, will only increase system imbalances in the long run. The diet that the majority of Americans follow is concentrated heavily in foods that deplete energy (soft drinks, sugar, milk and dairy products, potatoes, etc.) Vitamins only treat nutritional symptoms superficially. They do not get to the root of the problem. You may feel a little better for a few weeks, but then the symptoms return.

Taking vitamins increases the stress on your entire system by raising yang energy so high that it further depletes the yin energy your body needs to regain its equilibrium and vitality. Vitamins cause stress to the liver because it has to work two or three times as hard to eliminate and digest vitamin supplements properly. If the liver is too weak to do the job well, the residue of vitamins that cannot be utilized by the body will cause the body heat to rise (defense mechanism) and cause symptoms of constipation, headache, impatience, irritability, and dark yellow urine. Vitamins should not be necessary if you are eating foods that are balanced in energy for your constitution.

Salt

The popularity of macrobiotic cooking and the concern about hypertension and high blood pressure have wrought much confusion about salt. Extremes in position are not really necessary on this issue.

Salt is essential to survival. It is a basic ingredient in blood. It helps to strengthen vitality and mental clarity. The amount of salt needed is dependent on a person's age, health condition, activity level, and environmental conditions. Too much salt intake causes hyperactivity, irritability, kidney problems, thirstiness, and a tendency to anger easily, among other things. Too little salt causes poor circulation, mental lethargy, sleepiness, and weakness, for example. Salt creates yin energy, and eating too much can cause an imbalance that makes you crave yang foods, such as ice cream and other sweets, especially after you finish a meal. If used moderately and appropriately, salt can enhance food by drawing out its natural flavor and sweetness. Learning how to adjust salt intake and finding its balance with oil and water is an important part of the art of cooking.

The best kind of salt to use is white unrefined sea salt. It is richer in valuable trace elements than that which has been mined, washed, and kiln-dried.

The Importance of Enzymes

To understand and appropriately evaluate nutritional needs, one must recognize individual metabolic characteristics as well as system imbalances. In other words, it is not sufficient to know the vitamin / mineral needs of the body, but also the body's approach to absorbing and using what it receives.

Enzymes play a very important role in this process. They are the substances that make life possible because they are needed for every chemical reaction that occurs in the body. Without enzymes, there would be no food absorption or the conversion of food into energy. Their main function is to change food from one form to another. They assist in breaking it down so that it can dissolve and pass through the intestinal wall into the bloodstream, thus feeding the cells. Eating foods whose enzymes have been damaged through cooking too long or at very high heat, or eating combinations of food that do not complement each other enzymatically can literally cause you to "starve" from poor assimilation of vital nutrients.

All living foods contain enzymes, especially greens, sprouts, seeds, grains, fruits, and vegetables. In addition to serving as catalysts, enzymes give off a kind of energy when they work. They consist of protein carriers charged with energy factors just as a battery consists of metallic plates charged with electricity. Although they perform many astounding feats, they are easily destroyed by heat, cold, and acid foods.

PLANNING MEALS

To help you plan balanced and nutritious meals simply and quickly, I have included suggestions for foods, 7-day meal plans, alternative foods to try, and a form you can use in developing your own meals. These are all meant as a guide. Follow the principles you have learned and your own intuition for what is best for your life and body.

CHOOSING FOODS

On the following pages you will find foods in basic categories which I recommend you stock for either regular or occasional use. When making decisions about when to use which items, one helpful hint is to choose those that are grown locally and are in season. These will always have the advantage of containing energies most in keeping with nature's rhythms and will have the highest Qi essence of that food. You may, of course, include whatever foods are your family's favorites due to culture, religion, health, or condition (mental, emotional, or environmental.) The foods I have listed are just a guideline. There are not absolutes. Be as creative as you like.

FOODS FOR REGULAR USE

Grains: barley, basmati rice, brown rice (long grain or medium grain), millet, pearl barley, quinoa, rye, teff.

Vegetables: acorn squash, bean sprouts, black mushrooms, bok choy, broccoli, burdock, butternut squash, cabbage, carrots and their tops, cauliflower, chinese cabbage, collard greens, daikon and their tops, dandelion roots/leaves, hubbard squash, kale, kokkaido pumpkin, lima beans, lotus root, mustard greens, okra, parsley, peas, pumpkin, radishes, red cabbage, rutabaga, spinach, squash, turnip greens, watercress.

Legumes: adzuki beans, black soybeans, chickpeas, lentils, peas, soybeans.

Sea Vegetables: agar agar, arame, dulse, hijiki, irish moss, kombu, mekabu, toasted nori, wakame.

Pickles: bran pickle, pressed pickle, sauerkraut, takian pickle, tamari pickle.

Beverages: bancha stem tea, bancha twig tea, roasted barley tea, roasted brown rice tea, spring well water (if not available, use reverse osmosis water).

Seasonings and Oils: fish sauce, gamasio sesame salt, green onion, natural miso, natural soy sauce, sea vegetable powder, tamari sauce, umeboshi plum & paste, umeboshi vinegar, unrefined white sea salt.

Occasional Use
Grains: brown rice (short grain), corn, corn on the cob, red rice, sweet rice.

Fruit: seasonally and & locally grown.

Seeds and Nuts: almonds, cashews, chestnuts, peanuts, pumpkin seeds, sesame seeds, sunflower seeds, walnuts.

Seafood: clams, cod, flounder, halibut, lobster, oysters, red snapper, sole, trout, white meat fish in general.

Beverages: corn silk tea, dandelion tea, ginger tea, mu tea.

Seasonings and Oils: all kinds of pepper, cinnamon, dark or light sesame oil, ginger, horseradish, lemongrass/citronella root, mint, olive oil, rice vinegar, roasted sesame seed, safflower oil, saffron, thyme.

Snacks: left over noodles, left over rice, rice balls, rice cakes, roasted seeds, sushi.

Other: rice paper (tissue thin round sheet of dried rice paste which is sturdy enough to wrap things into a roll after it is dampened and softened with water)

Whenever possible, plan your meals in advance. When shopping, try to buy food for the entire week. Make sure you have plenty of the basics on hand (brown rice, sweet rice, beans, and dry noodles.) Buy only fresh foods, grains, vegetables, fruit, etc. Buy green vegetables to be eaten the first three days of the week since they will not stay fresh for long periods of time; purchase rooted or hearty vegetables to be eaten the last four days of the week. For example,

First part of the week: artichokes, broccoli, kale, mustard greens, spinach

Second part of the week: cabbage, corn, eggplant, mushrooms, potatoes, squash, tomatoes, zucchini.

Take advantage of the wide selection of delicious and healthy herbs available for use as seasoning. Fresh ginger, cumin, sage, and many others can be put to good use in your cooking. Be creative and have fun. Eating healthy doesn't have to be dull, boring, and tasteless.

The best all-around oil to stock is olive oil. If unavailable or too expensive, purchase the purest, cold-pressed oil available. Unsaturated vegetable oils such as those extracted from peanuts, corn, sesame seeds, and soybeans are recommended. Avoid hardened vegetable shortenings.

7-DAY MEAL PLANS

On the next two pages you will find two suggested 7-day diet plans, one for vegetarians, and one for meat-eaters. They are not tailored to every need and are not meant to be followed to the letter. They are only intended to serve as examples of how to combine foods and when to eat certain types of foods. You can refer to these charts as guidelines in planning your own diet and meals. If you have undertaken the quest to understand balance within your own body and life, you will want to continually experiment with the foods you feel are appropriate for you while using the principles outlined in this book.

Some people need more food than listed here; others will need less. Your age, body size, the climate you live in, the type of work you do, and your emotional state at the time you eat will all be contributing factors. If you need more food than recommended, add a piece of toast, an extra piece of fruit, or an additional vegetable. Feel free to combine menus to create meals that suit your own taste and health conditions. Also, use your common sense when deciding the proportions of each food to eat, so that you maintain an appropriate weight for you. The most important thing is to have three regular meals a day to keep your body operating efficiently.

Following the 7-day diet plans, you will find a blank planning form. I use this form in my clinical practice as a diagnostic tool and to help my patients become more aware of their current food intake. Many have given me an embarrassed look as they hand me the form and exclaim, "I

7-DAY DIET PLAN FOR VEGETARIANS

BREAKFAST	LUNCH	DINNER
(DAY 1) Whole grain toast Almond butter Cup of hot herbal tea	Cooked brown rice and adzuki beans* Steamed artichoke* Herbal tea	Baked potato Seaweed and onion soup* Baked vegetables*
(DAY 2) 7-grain cereal Glass of soy milk	Couscous salad* Steamed green beans	Miso soup* Cooked brown rice Blanched spinach Ginger tea / grapes
(DAY 3) Brown rice cereal Soy milk, tea, or wheat grass juice	Fettuccine sautéed with safflower oil Ratatouille	Grain salad* Mixed drink of Perrier, lime, and raw brown sugar
(DAY 4) Homemade granola* Soy milk Banana	Brown rice Sweet and sour eggplant* Steamed broccoli Watermelon	Baked butternut squash and onion* Artichoke spaghetti w/ sauce (no meat) Warm tea
(DAY 5) Whole grain toast Cashew butter Glass of soy milk or hot tea	Cooked brown rice with lentils* Gamisio* Green tea	Minestrone soup* Sesame seed crackers Avocado Hot tea
(DAY 6) Oatmeal with raisins Glass of soy milk or hot tea	Grain salad* Orange or nectarine Hot tea	Vegetable soup* Cooked brown rice Tofu and black mushrooms* Kiwi Lotus root tea
(DAY 7) 7-grain cereal Gamisio* Glass of soy milk or hot tea	Vegetable soup* with whole grain crackers Peaches Hot tea	Cooked brown rice and adzuki beans* Steamed artichoke* or alfalfa sprouts Sautéed tofu and zucchini Green tea

*these recipes can be found in the Recipe section.

7-DAY DIET PLAN FOR MEAT-EATERS

BREAKFAST	LUNCH	DINNER
(DAY 1) Sweet rice* Gamisio* Green tea or Wheat grass tea	Tuna sandwich with alfalfa sprouts Cucumbers and tomatoes Mixed drink of Perrier, lime, and raw brown sugar	Artichoke spaghetti with spaghetti sauce Steamed broccoli Warm tea
(DAY 2) Homemade granola* Soy milk Honeydew melon Toast	Bean salad* Warm tea	Stir-fried seafood and vegetables* Black bean soup* Chamomile tea Cooked brown rice
(DAY 3) Oatmeal with raisins Soy milk Green tea	Cooked brown rice Chicken breast with broccoli* Bojenmi tea	Shrimp with pineapple* Magnificent minestrone soup* Warm tea
(DAY 4) Whole grain toast Almond butter Banana Warm herbal tea	Kicheree* Green tea	Sesame rice* Steamed artichoke* Turkey soup* Warm tea
(DAY 5) Whole grain rye bread Omelet Wheat grass juice	Chicken salad* Whole grain crackers Warm tea	Baked potato Blanched spinach Pork chops and lemon grass* Warm tea
(DAY 6) 7-grain cereal with raisins Soy milk	Grain salad* Soy milk or ginger tea Watermelon	Cooked brown rice Steamed green beans Fish stew* Green tea
(DAY 7) Brown rice cereal Soy milk	Couscous salad* Orange or avocado Wheatgrass juice drink	Fettuccine with sweet and sour eggplant* Chicken with ginger* Sweet potato Chamomile tea

*these recipes can be found in the Recipe section.

7-DAY DIET FORM

BREAKFAST	LUNCH	DINNER
DAY 1		
DAY 2		
DAY 3		
DAY 4		
DAY 5		
DAY 6		
DAY 7		

can't believe what I ate last week! It's a good thing you had me write this down!" For this reason, I am including this form for you in your own self-evaluation. It is always best to become fully aware of your present dietary habits before making any changes. First, track your eating habits—everything you eat—for a week. Review the form at the end of the week in light of the balancing principles you have learned and your knowledge of your own constitution. You may be amazed by how much you vary from your ideal diet. Then, use the form to help you plan meals for the next seven days. Develop a diet that is more in harmony with your constitution, your activities, and the seasons. Most likely you will need to make changes, sometimes major, to your usual habits. These can happen slowly over time. But now you know your goal, and you can keep moving along the path and make adjustments at the pace you can manage.

BREAKFAST, LUNCH, AND DINNER— HELPFUL HINTS

I have compiled this section to give you some quick ideas when deciding what to eat for breakfast, lunch, or dinner. Some of the information is repeated from earlier sections of the book but should prove helpful as a quick review.

Breakfast
Breakfast is the most important meal of the day. The stomach energy is at its highest in the morning and is ready to fuel the body for the day ahead. Carbohydrates are what it needs most at that time. The more active and strenuous your day, the more carbohydrates you will need. The following choices are recommended for a hearty, nutritious breakfast.

- Rolled Oats: Cooked with spring water, this is an excellent morning carbohydrate to start a busy day.

- Oatmeal (unprocessed): Purchase raw oatmeal for a nutritious and fibrous food.

- Oat Bran: Quick to prepare and wholesome as well. It can be eaten with sesame seeds (gamisio) or raisins.

- Cream of Wheat / Cream of Rice

- Sweet Rice: Natural sweet rice makes a tasty breakfast, especially when topped with a pinch of sea salt, two pinches of raw sugar, and fresh ground nuts or baked sesame seeds.

- Whole Grain Toast: You can never go wrong with toast made from natural whole grain breads such as rye, wheat, and oatmeal. It is best to avoid or minimize high-fat dairy butter. Consider using almond butter, cashew butter, sesame butter, or peanut butter instead.

- Although unusual in America, any whole grain combined with nuts, beans, or a healthy meat will make a complete meal and a solid, healthy breakfast. Examples would be brown rice and lentils, red rice and adzuki beans.

- Avoid foods high in fat, sugar, and cholesterol. Eggs can be eaten occasionally—no more than two per week.

Lunch

During the day, people are all business and are always in a hurry. Eating alone or with friends is usually done at a sandwich shop or fast food restaurant. A business luncheon may offer more atmosphere but still consists of the usual high fat and rich cuisine. In my opinion, lunch is the second most important meal of the day and should be taken more seriously than it is. We must learn to be much kinder to our bodies during lunch to fuel ourselves for the rest of the day. The following are some guidelines for your lunch time meal.

- When eating out, order healthful entrees such as broiled, baked, or grilled fish, small portions of lean beef, or baked fowl.

- Choose baked or boiled potatoes or rice instead of french fries, chips, or the like.

- Select steamed or boiled vegetables over salads and cole slaw.

- Opt for whole grain breads or at least fresh baked bread or corn bread instead of white flour bread, biscuits, rolls, and hushpuppies.

- Try to order mineral water instead of the restaurant's tap water. Whatever you drink, order it without ice. If you need to be especially alert in the afternoon, avoid drinking beer or a cocktail.

- If you want to have a sandwich for lunch, order tuna fish or turkey on whole grain bread or toast. Feel free to add sprouts and tomatoes but avoid cheese and chips.

- Soups are also a good and nutritious lunch food if they are made from fresh ingredients. Avoid canned soups. Whole grain crackers are the perfect complement to soups and are healthy too.

- In general, stay with the freshest, least processed, and most healthful items on a menu. Use your common sense to help you make the right choice. It is best to pass on the dessert.

- If you are able to pack and bring your own lunch, follow the general rules for cooking and eating listed elsewhere in the guidebook. You can always eat leftovers from the previous night's dinner or pack one of the sandwiches mentioned above. Also, keep bottled or mineral water on hand at work rather than resorting to tap water, coffee, or soft drinks.

Dinner

Contrary to popular belief, dinner is not the most important meal of the day. In fact, it is the least important and should be as light as possible. Your body is winding down for the day and preparing to rest and cleanse itself during the nighttime hours.

A big heavy dinner adversely affects this process. If you do eat a heavy dinner, try to finish before 7:00 PM so that your stomach can do most of its hard work while you are still awake and active. Vegetables usually take a few hours to be fully digested, but meat takes from twelve to eighteen hours. Therefore, eating mostly vegetables at dinner and eating meat earlier in the day is a good practice. In general, though, eating late will distress the body and may cause bad dreams or nightmares.

Try to combine your foods in compatible, complementary ways. Rice, beans, unbleached pasta, healthful noodles, and whole grains are recommended at dinner time. Here are some additional tips:

- Brown rice should become a mainstay in your diet. It is extremely healthy, contains fiber, and is a foundation food for combination with many other foods. It will keep you grounded and centered.

- For meats, stick to fish, seafood, veal, lamb, pork, and lean beef. I personally do not recommend chicken unless it is kosher. Kosher chicken contains less contaminants than most supermarket birds. Chicken should be either grilled, baked, or broiled.

- Lightly steam or boil your vegetables in order to retain the maximum amount of vitamins and minerals.

- Avoid frying your foods. Frying food removes natural vitamins and fried foods create excess body heat as you try to digest them.

- Remember not to drink with your meals. Always drink thirty minutes before or two hours after meals.

COOKING METHODS

One way to achieve dynamic and healthy eating is to vary cooking and preserving methods. You can alternate the following methods for pleasing results:

REGULAR METHODS	OCCASIONAL METHODS
Pressure cooking	Sautéing
Boiling	Stir-frying
Steaming	Serving raw food
Waterless cooking	Deep frying
Making soups	Making tempura
Pickling	Baking
Oil-less sautéing (w/water)	
Pressing	

The methods in the first column can be alternated regularly. Those in the second column should be incorporated only occasionally.

Other ways you can achieve variety and interest are by: (1) different ways of cutting vegetables, (2) using different amounts of water, (3) varying the amount and kind of seasoning, (4) changing the length of cooking time, and (5) using higher or lower heat.

COOKWARE AND UTENSILS NEEDED

Simplicity is important in living a quality life. To maintain the proper relationship with our food and its preparation, we should reconsider the need for many of our modern utensils. These were developed as we complicated our food intake and alienated ourselves from food as an important element in nourishing our spirits. A modern kitchen encourages "living in the fast lane" and encumbers our spirits with many useless activities that actually keep us away from the joy waiting to be experienced through more balanced food intake. We must return to our former simplicity, not only to make our lives easier, but also to help us maintain a reverent attitude toward food preparation and assure the efficient assimilation of nutrients.

A significant consideration is the type of stove to use. Microwave cooking is not recommended at all. It zaps food with waves at three billion cycles per second, whereas an electric stove runs at only 60 cycles per second. A disadvantage of electric cooking, however, is that heating elements take too long to heat up or cool down. Additionally, electricity disintegrates the molecular structure and strength of food by causing the electrons to bounce out of the atomic field, leaving the atom very unstable. Because of this, you may not feel satisfied after your meal and could develop a strong craving for salt or animal food. Gas is a good cooking method because it does less damage to the molecules in the food.

The following is a list of other useful items for a kitchen; these encourage the maintenance of a simple, convenient, and pleasurable relationship between you and the preparation of your food. Keep in mind that the more simply you live, the fewer utensils you will need. You will not require all the items listed; choose those that are comfortable for you. These are just suggestions for those who need a little guidance.

- a stainless steel pressure cooker
- a baking container for bread (avoid aluminum)

- a wok

- several stainless steel mixing bowls in different sizes for washing and mixing food.

- a large wooden serving bowl for grain

- a stainless steel or bamboo steamer

- a colander for rinsing noodles and other food

- a fine strainer

- a muffin tin (avoid aluminum)

- a mortar and pestle (Crushing things often brings out the flavor more than chopping and grinding them. If you prefer a lighter weight, buy wood instead of stone.)

- a food mill for puréeing squash and other foods

- a teapot or kettle (avoid aluminum)

- a tea strainer

- large glass jars for storing grains, beans, nuts, seeds, etc.

- wooden cutting boards, one for fish or animal food, one for vegetables

- knives (stainless steel)

- a bread knife

- a grater for fresh ginger, daikon, carrots, etc.

- a vegetable peeler

- an oil skimmer

- a natural bristle brush for brushing oil into skillet

- a vegetable brush

- a wooden spoon for stirring, mixing, and scooping

- a bamboo rice paddle for serving grain

- soup ladles

- a rubber spatula for scraping pureed food

- a metal spatula for turning food over

- a cooking chopstick (longer than usual chopstick)

- a rolling pin

- measuring cups and spoons

- a sushi mat for making sushi

- cotton cheesecloth

- paper towels

- a skillet (a medium size measuring 8–10″ is preferred)

- pots (a 2-quart or 3-quart pot is good for soups)

THE CLOROX™ BATH FOR FRESH FOODS

Almost all meats and fruits and vegetables have been affected by pesticides, sprays, germs, fungus, and metallics. There are also many parasites that live in our soils and to which our bodies can become host. Many seemingly incurable conditions such as cancer may have their origins in the concentration of such substances in our systems. Washing all fresh foods is a necessary practice.

Use a Clorox™ bath to wash all fresh food. This will neutralize the deleterious effects of all outside invaders. Not only will this bath kill the eggs of many parasites and help to remove harmful toxins, it will also enhance the flavors of both fruits and vegetables and help them to stay fresher longer. We have all seen evidence in the media that the dangers from sprays and other materials used in so many ways in the processing of food may be greater than we know. Following the few simple steps outlined above will insure greater protection for your family.

Clorox™ Bath Formula:

- ½ tsp. of Clorox™ to 1 gallon of water

- Only use Clorox™, no other product seems to work as well.

- Do not use more Clorox™ than instructed.

- Do not leave fruits and vegetables in longer than the given time. Green leafy vegetables, in particular, will turn brown because of oxidation.

Fruits and Vegetables

- Thin-skinned fruits (such as berries, peaches, apricots, and plums) and vegetables require 10 minutes.

- Rooted vegetables and heavy-skinned fruits (such as apples, all citrus fruit, and bananas) require 15–20 minutes.

Timing is very important! Make a fresh bath for each group. After the Clorox™ bath, place fruits and vegetables in a fresh water bath for 10–15 minutes.

Eggs

The egg shell is porous and can absorb pesticide sprays, causing allergic reactions in many people. Salmonella bacteria may also be present. By bathing eggs in a Clorox™ for 20–30 minutes, the amount of salmonella bacteria will be greatly reduced, the eggs will have a better flavor, and there will be a reduction in their tendency to create allergies.

Meat and Fish

Meats are another major category of food requiring bathing. In addition to bacteria, meat can carry chemicals from injections or toxins from animal feed. All flesh foods (excluding ground meat) and fish, which carries a heavy mercury content, should be placed in a Clorox™ bath for 10–15 minutes (for a 2 to 5 lb. weight). The flavor will be improved, the tissue tenderized, and toxic substances neutralized. Frozen turkey or chicken should remain in the Clorox™ bath until thawed.

selecting food

Eating for Balance and Harmony

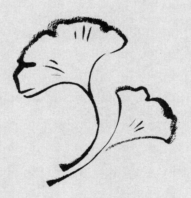

THE BASIC FOODS

Whole grains, legumes, seeds, and nuts are the most important and potent health-building foods. These foods should be the basic components of any healthy diet. Their nutritional value is unsurpassed by any other food. Eaten raw or cooked, they contain balanced combinations of all the important nutrients essential for human growth, sustenance of health, and prevention of disease. In addition, they contain the secret of life itself, the germ, the reproductive power that assures the perpetuation of each species. This reproductive power, the spark of life in all seeds, is of extreme importance for the life, health, and reproductive ability of human beings.

The foods in these basic groups are excellent sources of proteins. They are also the best natural sources of essential unsaturated fatty acids, without which health cannot be maintained. They are nature's best source of lecithin, a substance that is invaluable to the healthful functioning of the brain, nerves, glands (especially sex glands), and arteries.

The vitamin content of grains, legumes, seeds, and nuts is unsurpassed. They are an especially great source of vitamin E and B-complex vitamins. Vitamin E is vital for the preservation of health and prevention of premature aging. And B-complex vitamins are essential for practically all body functions. They are very much involved in protecting the body against stress. They are particularly needed by the hypoglycemic; they are directly involved in sugar metabolism and the sugar control mechanisms. A deficiency of vitamin B can damage the adrenal cortex, which is often at the root of low blood sugar problems.

Grains, legumes, seeds, and nuts are also gold mines of minerals and trace elements. More and more research is showing that minerals are even more important to health than the more glamorized vitamins. A balanced body chemistry, especially in terms of acidity and alkalinity, is dependent on minerals. Biochemical disorder in the system, of which sugar metabolism is one process, is a basic underlying cause of most disease.

The foods in these groups contain other very beneficial nutrients: pacifarins, an antibiotic resistance factor that increases man's natural resistance to disease; and zuxones, which produce vitamins in the body, play a part in the rejuvenation of cells, and prevent premature aging.

Recently, the benefits of the bulk and roughage content of whole grains, legumes, seeds, and nuts, have brought their importance back into the public focus. After several decades of eating refined and processed foods, from which the outer coating, the bulk, has been processed out, man has become plagued with constipation, diverticulitis, colitis, and cancer of the colon. Current studies show that to avoid this epidemic, we must go back to whole, unprocessed grains, seeds, legumes, and nuts in order to provide the bulk necessary to prevent these disorders.

WHOLE GRAINS

Listed below are several of the most popular grains throughout the world. For each I present information on their nutritional value and their beneficial application for certain dietary deficiencies.

All grains and legumes should be cooked or sprouted. Sprouting breaks down phytin and releases minerals, thus increasing the nutritive value of the original grain, legume, seed, or nut. Refined polished grains should be avoided altogether.

Rice

For thousand of years, rice has been the staple food of over half the world. The Chinese in particular consider rice the main food for humans. They have learned from centuries of experience that the triple burner is where the Qi flow starts and ends and is also the pathway of water and grain. Rice, a neutral food, has the effect of harmonizing the yin and yang balance of the body—a state needed to maintain good health. Therefore, it is an important staple food that ideally should be included in each meal, or at least in one meal a day.

Rice is a bulk food relatively low in calories as compared with other food normally eaten in American diets. Compare, for example, the following items:

$3\frac{1}{2}$ oz (100 gms.) of cooked rice contain only 109 calories
$3\frac{1}{2}$ slices of white bread contain 269 calories
$3\frac{1}{2}$ rolls contain 339 calories

Rice can be a very good substitute for potato chips, breads, potatoes, rolls, stuffing, cereals, cookies, biscuits, and other starchy foods. Because of its high bulk, it satisfies hunger quickly and is easily digested when prepared properly (without adding butter, oil, salt, gravy, or sauce.) It is low in fat and sodium and free of cholesterol. It contains all eight of the essential amino acids. It is superior in this respect to all other grains. It also provides thiamin B_1, riboflavin B_2, and niacin B_3,—vitamins that are essential for the normal functioning of the brain and muscles.

Rice in combination with legumes is a source of meatless protein. The amino acids in rice can be very effectively used by your body as a "building block" to create tissues and regulate body processes. Rice contains very little of the amino acids isoleucine and lysine. Yet in combination with legumes, which are high in the content of these amino acids, rice will contribute in forming complete proteins. It is also rich in the mineral molybdenum, which is important for proper carbohydrate metabolism.

Rice plays an important role in Chinese cuisine for its aesthetic, as well as its nutritional advantages. Its light color is a dramatic contrast to other foods. Its blandness clears the palate and accents the flavor of even the most simple vegetable.

All whole grain rice is referred to as "brown rice." There is short grain and long grain brown rice. Short grain contains less protein, more minerals, and is heavier and more starchy than long grain. Therefore, long grain is preferable for regular use. Brown rice will not be as tender as white rice because the nutrient-rich bran layer tends to remain firm after cooking.

Preparation

Brown rice takes a little more time to cook than white rice. Use two cups of brown rice with $3\frac{1}{2}$ cups of water. Bring the water to a boil, add the rice, and cook until the water and rice come to the same level, or until it is heavy when you stir it. It may take 10–15 minutes to boil. Then turn the heat to medium low for another 15–20 minutes. It will take from 30 to 45 minutes to cook brown rice, depending on the amount you use.

Adding lentils, barley, or millet is a great way to enhance the flavor. You can use half of one and half of another. I do not recommend, however, adding butter, gravy, salt, or oil to the rice. When you keep rice plain with its own flavor, it is easier distinguish the flavors of the dishes you are preparing to combine with it. Ordinarily, one would not eat rice by itself. It is usually served with stir-fried vegetables or boiled fish. It is advisable to make fresh rice every day.

Wheat

Wheat is very popular in this country and is a component of almost every product on the supermarket shelves. It can be beneficial to the liver and help young people to develop their muscles and endurance. Wheat, however, is very rich in gluten, a substance that causes aches and pains in joints and vaginal discharge, especially if eaten every day. It also can cause inflammation if body resistance has become weak. Also, because of its excessive consumption in American diets, most Americans have developed allergies to wheat.

Recent anthropological research has revealed that evidence of arthritic conditions does not appear in human skeletal remains until about the same time that wheat began being cultivated by humans. This may yet be inconclusive; however, oriental medicine has recognized wheat's adverse effects on joints for centuries. Use your own judgment when cooking with wheat. It would be advisable to avoid it when trying to heal an inflamed wound or get rid of a cold because it is mucus-forming.

I do not recommend purchasing whole wheat bread, because whole wheat flour can go rancid very easily. The oil in the wheat germ causes whole wheat flour to become rancid far more quickly than white flour, which has the germ removed. This is why products made with white flour have a longer shelf life than those made with whole wheat flour. If you do buy whole wheat bread, make sure to get it from a bakery that grinds its own flour; that way there is less chance that the flour is old or rancid.

Barley

Barley is one of my favorite grains. It originated in North Africa and Southeast Asia and is rich in vitamins and minerals. It stimulates the liver and the lymphatic system and is therefore excellent for eliminating mucus. Pearl barley has had most of its vitamins and minerals removed during milling, but it is beneficial for weak and sick people because it's easily digestible.

Oats

Oats are a yin grain, especially nourishing the yin essence. I recommend this grain to many of my patients. It is my usual breakfast.

Oats are high in assimilable calcium. They are beneficial for all types of nervous irritations and debilities. For this reason, oats are one of the finest foods to use in convalescent environments. Also, eating oatmeal regularly helps in developing resistance to weather related arthritic and rheumatic complaints.

Oats are beneficial to those women who suffer from menstrual cramps. Oriental practitioners consider it to have a neutralizing effect on reproductive and sexual systems. It has also proven of great benefit to pregnant and nursing mothers.

Finally, oats are quickly and easily prepared. Try to buy the finest whole oats instead of processed instant oatmeal.

Corn

Very popular in America, corn helps build strong blood and strengthens the heart. But it is the least nutritionally complete grain. Corn is best eaten with beans or other foods to guarantee a complete meal.

Millet

Millet is alkaline in nature and toning for the spleen and stomach. Mild to digest, it is a good breakfast for children and older people. It makes a great soup when cooked with barley and beans.

LEGUMES

Legumes are one of the earliest crops cultivated by man. Even in Biblical times legumes were known for their nutritional value. They should be a staple in your diet as a main source of protein. In fact, the protein in some legumes is equal to or greater than that in meat. I recommend using lentils, peas, black beans, and soybeans to make delicious satisfying soups.

Preparation

Beans need to soak overnight. If you forget to soak them, bring them to a boil in a pot and discard the water. Add fresh water and cook in a pressure cooker until soft. Add vegetables and tamari or salt after the beans become soft. You may want to save leftover liquid from boiling the vegetables to use in making soup. You can add your choice of vegetable, fish flakes, seaweed, dried mushrooms, and a whole grain. (See the recipe section for more specific instructions on preparing delicious meals with legumes.)

SEEDS

As people become more health conscious, many are eating lighter meals, changing to a vegetarian regimen, or avoiding milk and other dairy products. Consequently, there is a lot of concern about how to get enough calcium. In looking for alternatives, many have discovered the nutritional value of seeds. I have listed a few of the most popular seeds here. There are many more you can find. Experiment with all of them to find those that suit your taste and health condition. I am sure you will find that including a variety of seeds or nuts in your daily diet for snacking is fun, economical, and enhances your health.

Sesame Seeds

In Japan and other oriental countries like Vietnam, Singapore, and Korea, sesame seeds play an important part in cooking and baking. George Oshawa, a leader in macrobiotic research for fifteen years, believes that a person cannot only survive on brown rice and sesame seeds but can actually maintain optimum health and cure many diseases.

Nutritionally, sesame seeds are a powerhouse. They contain over thirty-five percent protein and have twice as much calcium as milk. They also contain as much phosphorous, niacin, and thiamin as liver meat. Finally, they contain between forty to sixty percent oil, an oil that is prized not only for its flavor but also its ability to resist oxidation and rancidity. It is best to buy chemically free, hulled sesame seeds.

Sunflower Seeds

Sunflower seeds are a nutritious seed as well. They are lower in protein, phosphorous, and calcium than sesame seeds. They are, however, high in vitamins D, E, and B-complex. They also contain a trace of flourine, which is beneficial for teeth. Sunflower seeds make a delicious snack or can be toasted and added to a salad.

Pumpkin Seeds

Pumpkin seeds contain up to twenty-nine percent protein and play an important part in the diet of both North and South America, India, and some countries in Southeast Asia. They are beneficial in treating prostrate gland problems. They are nutritious for snacking, in cereals, or toasted and sprinkled on salads.

HERBS

In many Southeast Asian countries, herbs are used for their cleansing properties as well as for their ability to enhance the taste of food. They detoxify the blood by cleansing our systems from toxins in foods such as beef, pork, fish, and chicken.

Herbs such as ginger, cumin, red pepper, cayenne pepper, black and white pepper, rosemary, thyme, curry, sage, anise, and turmeric are very important in oriental cooking.

The following is a list of herbs commonly used in homes for their medicinal properties. You should stock them and keep them handy. It is better to know a few herbs that are useful and practical for everyday use, and to know them well, than it is to know too many and not be able to use them effectively. (See the home remedy section for the medicinal applications of many of these herbs.)

Ginger

Ginger is a stimulant. It is used to warm up the stomach and is one of the most effective digestants in the herbal kingdom. It is often very helpful in the treatment of colic (a stomach disorder). It also improves circulation and enhances the blood value.

Ginger can be made into a tea for daily use. It is especially good to drink in the winter and during menstruation. Use ginger when cooking with chicken, beef, and fish. It has a tonifying effect when added to bean sprouts, black beans, and red beans.

Parsley

Parsley is rich in vitamins A and C, with a good dose of vitamin B. It contains four times more vitamin A than carrots. It is also rich in calcium, copper, iron, and manganese, which all help to tonify the blood. As an herb tea, it has been helpful in treating gallstones and kidney stones. Eaten at the end of a meal, it freshens the breath. Its chlorophyll content helps wash away any hard onion, garlic, or fish odors.

Sage

Sage helps to reduce mucus and secretions. It aids in treating congestion in the respiratory passages. It can alleviate night sweating. It can also help reduce the milk of a mother who has just weaned her child. Sage also has disinfectant and astringent qualities. Crushed sage leaves are a useful first aid for insect bites. Tea made from sage is beneficial as an antiseptic gargle for a sore. Caution, however, must be exercised in using sage. Toxicity can develop with overconsumption.

Thyme

Thyme is useful in treating coughs, bronchitis, diarrhea, chronic gastritis, and flatulence. It is also useful in treating bruises, sprains, and rheumatic problems. Pregnant women should avoid fresh thyme, it acts strongly on the reproductive organs and could induce a miscarriage. Thyme has an active ingredient called thymol which is used in mouthwash, toothpaste, and to expel hookworms.

Cumin

Cumin seed stimulates the appetite and helps digestion.

Coriander

Coriander seed helps digestion and cools the body heat.

Cloves

Cloves have antiseptic properties and can be used in relieving toothache pain. Made into a tea, it can be effectively used to relieve flatulence.

Cinnamon

Cinnamon is often used by oriental practitioners in combination with other herbs to check a fever. It is particularly good to use in the winter to help ward off cold from the elements.

Saffron

Saffron is a rich flower, which can be used to keep a cold in check.

Turmeric

Turmeric is an excellent preservative, which can also be used as an antiseptic.

Fennel

Fennel seed is useful as an eyewash to strengthen eyesight and relax tired eyes.

Corn Silk

Corn silk is effective in treating bladder infections.

Castor Oil

Castor oil, applied alternatively with the juice of fresh cranberries, will remove corns or warts.

SPECIAL FOODS AND ORIENTAL FOODS

Many traditional oriental foods have very high nutritional value which cannot easily be found in foods common to the American diet. In making your transition to full health and vitality, I encourage you to consider including some of these special foods in your meals. This chapter includes background information which will help you become more familiar with these foods and assist you in learning to purchase and prepare them.

SEAWEED

Seaweeds are a nutritional and vitamin power source. As a food group, seaweed ranks second in calcium and phosphorous content, and first in magnesium, iron, iodine, and sodium. It contains up to twenty-five percent more protein than milk, while remaining naturally low in calories due to its low fat content. In addition, it contains vitamins A, B,

C, D$_3$, E, and K and fructose, an easily digestible sugar. Most importantly, seaweed is rich in vitamin B$_{12}$, which is needed for the proper functioning of the neuromuscular system.

The mineral and alkaline effects of seaweed purify the blood by eliminating the acid effects of a modern diet. Seaweed also helps dissolve fat and mucus deposits. Due to its vitamin B$_{12}$ content, it is helpful in treating and avoiding pernicious anemia.

I highly recommend adding seaweed to your daily diet whether you are a meat-eater or a vegetarian. It is difficult to find a more nutritious food which acts like a natural vitamin supplement. For those who begin to eat seaweed and don't like the taste of fish, try the mild tasting seaweeds such as dulse, kombu, arame, and nori. Kelp, wakame, and hijiki have a stronger flavor. You may want to introduce seaweed to your cooking slowly, one kind at a time. If you and your family don't like it, don't give up. Put it aside and try it again another day or another week. It may seem strange to you at first because you have never been exposed to it before. But give yourself some time. Eventually, you can grow to really like it.

Preparation and Storage

Seaweeds are dry when purchased. They need to be soaked with enough water to allow for expansion. Hijiki expands a lot more than arame. Retain the soaking water for use in recipes if possible. Pour carefully from the soaking bowl and discard the last part as it may contain sand particles.

Sea vegetables are great for long-term storage as long as you keep them in air-tight jars after opening their packages. If they become damp, simply dry briefly in the oven on low heat or in the sun. White spots that may appear on their surface are crystals of salt that have formed due to changes in temperature.

Arame, Wakame, Hijiki

To prepare arame, wakame, and hijiki: Wash seaweed quickly. Cover and soak in water for 10 minutes. Sauté one thinly sliced onion and one slivered carrot in sesame oil. Add the seaweed and simmer for 30–40 minutes. Season with soy sauce to taste.

Kombu

I personally like using kombu in rice to add flavor and color. Soak kombu with water for 5 minutes. Add to the rice when it is boiling. Kombu can also be eaten as a separate dish.

Dulse

Dulse makes an excellent snack. Chew a little piece at a time or sprinkle it on soups.

Nori

Nori is most known for its use in sushi rolls, but can be exceptional in soups as well. It has a mild flavor and is one of the richest sea vegetable sources of protein. It also contains large amounts of vitamin C and B_1 and is especially rich in vitamin A.

Nori is usually sold dried as ten 7-inch square sheets folded in a package. Sheet nori varies considerably in both price and quality. A good grade nori will have an overall green translucence with an even texture when held up to the light. Cheaper grades will be purple, limp, and uneven. They may also be artificially dyed green and chemically lacquered.

TOFU

Tofu is a staple food in any vegetarian diet. It is made from soybeans and for centuries has been a primary food of millions of people throughout Asia. Tofu contains high quality protein, no cholesterol, is very low in calories, and is very inexpensive to buy and make. For variety in flavor and texture, I recommend three ways to use tofu. The first and primary method is to use fresh tofu on its own or add it to almost any cooked dish.

A second method is to freeze the package of tofu. The process of freezing will add air pockets to the tofu and toughen it. It then becomes sponge-like in texture and chewy. It can be added to any soup or baked dish or stir-fried with vegetables. It can also be used as a base ingredient in vegetable burgers.

The third way to use tofu is to purchase fresh, firm-textured tofu and bake it. Place half-inch thick slabs directly onto your oven grill or a baking sheet and bake at 350 degrees for 20 minutes, or until golden yellow in color. This can be eaten as is or added to any cooked dish. This method can replace deep-fried tofu, which I do not recommend. Deep frying will raise the body's heat and may cause body system imbalances.

Tofu can be kept for a week or more under refrigeration if it is kept in water-filled containers and the water is changed daily. When tofu begins to have a slightly sour smell, it is starting to go bad. You can use it in a baking recipe immediately, or else discard the odorous batch. Tofu can be purchased in a vacuum sealed package which extends the life substantially.

TEMPEH

Tempeh is a traditional vegetarian product derived from fermenting soybeans. Its use originated in Indonesia. Tempeh is produced by a natural culturization process wherein soybeans are cultured with a mold called rhizopus oligosprus. Tempeh is rich in riboflavin, niacin, and vitamin B_6. It is also the richest vegetarian source of naturally occurring vitamin B_{12}. The protein found in tempeh is partially broken down during the fermentation process, which makes it easily digestible. For this reason, I highly recommend tempeh for children, weak, and elderly people.

SEITAN (WHEAT GLUTEN)

Seitan is a protein product made from wheat. By combining the protein-rich wheat flour with water and kneading the dough several times, the starch is removed from the flour. After cooking, seitan has a chewy texture similar to meat. Seitan is very high in protein and is used in a variety of ways in vegetarian cooking.

SOY SAUCE

Shoyu and tamari are Japanese names for natural soy sauce. Shoyu is fermented from soybeans, wheat, sea salt, and water. Tamari contains just soybeans, sea salt, and water. Shoyu is best for daily use because it has a richer flavor and is cheaper. Tamari is thicker, more mellow, and more expensive and is usually used for special dips and sauces. Always read labels carefully to know what you are buying.

MISO

Miso is a rich brown puree of soybeans fermented with sea salt. A cereal grain is usually added to it during processing. Miso is a complete and readily assimilable protein, which contains a good balance of carbohydrates, fats, minerals, and vitamins. It strengthens the digestive system and improves assimilation of carbohydrates. Like soy sauce and tamari, miso usually contains about twenty percent salt. So eat only small amounts of it each day.

Among the different kinds of miso available, two are predominant: barley miso (mugi miso) is suitable for daily use; and brown rice miso (genmai miso) is suitable for summer cooking. Both kinds contain small quantities of B_{12}, which is naturally produced during fermentation. Be sure to look for a brand which has been made with natural soy sauce. In general, miso makes an excellent soup base.

NUOC MAM (FISH SAUCE)

Nuoc Mam, originating in Vietnam, is used like salt or soy sauce in many oriental recipes. It is made with fish and, unlike salt or soy sauce, is a good source of protein. It is almost clear, with a slightly yellowish tint, and has a mild fishy odor. In Vietnam, Korea, and Thailand it is used as a basic seasoning for numerous dishes. You can find it in most oriental food store.

BLACK MUSHROOMS

Dried black mushrooms are very common in oriental foods, especially in vegetarian dishes. They add flavor and protein to your diet. You can purchase them at most oriental food stores or health food stores.

To cook dried black mushrooms, soak them first for 15 minutes until they soften. Then cut the stems off and discard. Slice the mushrooms into ⅛-inch thick pieces and add to casseroles, stir-fry, or other vegetable dishes.

OYSTER SAUCE

Made from oysters, oyster sauce is added as a thickener to many Chinese dishes. It is used in place of soy sauce or salt.

BEAN THREAD

Bean thread is a white thin noodle that is made from mung beans. It is gentle on the digestion and is less allergenic than egg or wheat noodles. Bean thread has a more chewy consistency than noodles and can be used in soups or in stir-fried dishes with vegetables.

CONGEE (OR CHÁO)

Congee is a very important food in Vietnam and many East Asian countries. It is highly prized for its use in strengthening the

Qi and blood. It is also useful in helping to reduce the build-up of summer heat in the body. It is easily digested and is a traditional remedy for strengthening the digestive system. In conjunction with other herbs, it can help to boost the immune system and improve circulation.

The main ingredient in congee is rice. Since rice is a diuretic, eating rice congee will help eliminate the toxins that build up in our bodies every day. See the section on "Healing with Food" for directions on congee's use for specific health conditions.

ALTERNATIVE FOODS FOR A HEALTHY DIET

As you progress along your path toward more healthful eating and nutrition, I urge you to begin to reduce your consumption of some foods, such as sodas, milk, butter, and wheat. This section will give you a number of interesting and tasty ideas for alternatives. Give them a try. I think you may be surprised how good these substitutes taste and make you feel. You may like them better than the original food!

ALTERNATIVES FOR TEAS, SODAS, COLD DRINKS, AND HOT BEVERAGES

Look at the supply of herbs and spices you have. Many of them, in their whole form, can be steeped and made into a delicious drink. Some good examples are:

- anise star

- cinnamon sticks

- ginger root

- licorice root
- sage leaf
- vanilla bean
- whole nutmeg or clove

ALTERNATIVES FOR SALT

Use these herbs alone or in combination: anise seed, basil, celery seed, clove, coriander, cumin, garlic, lemon peel, lemon-thyme, marjoram, oregano, pepper, rosemary, sage, sassafras, savory, and tarragon. Also, you can use soy sauce, tamari, shoyu, and fish sauce.

ALTERNATIVES FOR MILK AND CHEESE

- almond milk
- any nut milk
- goat's milk cheese or yogurt (can make yourself)
- sesame milk
- soy cheese
- soy milk
- soy yogurt
- sunflower milk
- tofu
- walnut milk

Milks can be made by blending nuts or seeds with water until a desired consistency is achieved.

ALTERNATIVES FOR BUTTER

Many butters can be purchased in health food stores or made by blending nuts or seeds with a little of the oil of the same nuts or seeds until the desired consistency is achieved.

- almond butter
- any nut butter
- apple butter
- bean dips
- cashew butter
- peanut butter
- pumpkin seed butter
- sunflower butter
- tahini (sesame butter)
- tofu spread
- vegetable dips

ALTERNATIVES FOR NOODLES

- bean noodles
- brown rice
- cauliflower
- eggplant
- green beans
- mung bean sprouts
- other whole grains

- potatoes
- tapioca
- tofu
- whole grain barley
- whole grain rye

ALTERNATIVES FOR DRESSINGS

- cooked beans, blended
- nuts or seeds, blended
- soft cheese, blended
- tofu, blended
- yogurt, blended
- lemon juice and oil
- lime juice, orange, or grapefruit juice
- vinegar and oil

ALTERNATIVES FOR SWEETENERS

- barley malt
- beet sugar
- date sugar
- fig
- fructose (corn syrup)
- herbs: angelica, balm, cardamom, chicory, cicely, licorice, miracle fruit, mint, and polypody

- honey
- lactose (milk sugar)
- molasses
- pure maple syrup
- rice syrup
- sorghum

ALTERNATIVES FOR GRAINS

- barley
- buckwheat
- chickpeas (garbanzo beans)
- corn
- corn meal
- cracked white corn
- millet
- oats
- potato flour
- rye
- soy flour, soy grits
- sweet potato flour
- sweet rice flour (mochiko)
- tapioca
- yam flour

ALTERNATIVE OILS

- almond
- apricot
- avocado
- cod liver
- corn
- mustard
- olive
- peanut
- pecan
- rice bran
- safflower
- sesame
- soy
- sunflower
- walnut

ALTERNATIVES FOR THICKENING AGENTS

- acacia gum
- agar agar
- arrowroot
- corn starch
- guar gum

- karaya gum
- legume flours
- lotus flour
- other grain flours
- rice flour (mochiko)
- sweet potato flour
- tapioca
- yam flour

ALTERNATIVES FOR EGGS IN BAKING

- arrowroot (1 tsp./egg)
- boiled flaxseed (1 glop/egg)
- sweet rice flour (1 tsp./egg)
- yam flour (1 tsp./egg)

healing with food

Preparing Remedies When You Are Sick

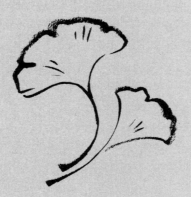

NATURAL HOME REMEDIES

In Chinese medicine, food is considered a healing tool because of the natural energy essence which it contains. Practitioners developed remedies over thousands of years by carefully observing the energetic effects of foods and herbs upon the energy patterns of people with various health conditions. They found that food energies can be used to counteract and balance energy patterns manifesting as illnesses. Many recipes can be easily prepared and used to treat minor ailments. Learning to routinely apply the appropriate foods to correct minor imbalances in yourself or your loved ones can help you avoid many extremes of poor health and the costly medical bills that evolve from them.

The natural home remedies described should not be considered "cure-alls." Some people will respond to these remedies better than others. If you have been polluting your body with denatured food substances on a regular basis for a long time, you may not respond as rapidly to natural remedies as someone who has been on a cleansing program for a while. Please consult with your healthcare practitioner to make sure a remedy is right for you and fits within your overall treatment plan.

Abdominal distention

- 3 ounces fresh peas, 3 cups fresh water. Blend together and drink twice a day.

Anemia or condition of weakness after recovering from an illness

- 5 ounces minced lean beef, 2 slices fresh ginger, a pinch of salt, or some soy sauce. Boil for 10 minutes in 1½ cups water. Eat the broth with rice twice a day.

- 10 ounces lamb, 1 ounce sliced fresh ginger, 2 cloves chopped garlic. Boil in 5 cups water until reduced to half. Add watercress or spinach. Eat with rice two to three times a day.

- 1 pound squid, 4 ounces black beans, ½ ounce ginger, a pinch of salt, 2 cups water. Boil for 1 hour on medium heat. Eat twice a day.

Appetite - poor

- Eat 4 ounces fresh cherries or drink 4 fluid ounces cherry juice before eating main meals.

- Eat 2 apricots two or three times a day or drink 4 fluid ounces apricot juice.

- 6 ounces barley, 3 ounces raw brown sugar, 2 cups water. Cook until reduced to half. Drink liquid while still lukewarm. Repeat every other day.

Asthma

- Drink juice from 5 ounces of fresh figs two times a day.

- Crush 3 cloves of garlic in one cup hot water. Drink two times a day.

Arteriosclerosis

- 3 ounces kelp, 4 ounces raw lean beef, 2 cups water. Cook until reduced to half. Eat every other day, including the broth.

Back pain - low back

- 3 ounces fresh crushed walnuts, 6 ounces raw brown sugar, 4 fluid ounces warm rice wine. Mix and drink twice a day for one month.

- 4 ounces mussels, 4 ounces lean pork, 2 cloves chopped garlic, 2 potatoes cut into small pieces, 2 cups water. Cook for 20 minutes. Eat twice a day, every other day for several weeks.

- Take 7 fresh chestnuts and dry them in an oven or under a grill, but do not brown them. Eat twice a day. Continue for 1 or 2 months.

Bee or wasp sting

- Mash a ripe banana and apply to the site of the sting.

Bladder infection

- First, avoid fried foods, coffee, chocolate, sugar, and hot spicy foods.

- Boil 3 ounces dried corn silk in 2 cups of water until reduced to half. Drink as a tea 4 to 5 times a day.

- Drink diluted cranberry juice throughout the day.

- Eat watermelon throughout the day (contains natural sulfur).

- Other foods that can help this condition are barley soup, chicken soup, and steamed vegetables.

Blood platelets - insufficient

- Drink 1 ounce red grape wine three times a day.

Boils

- Mash raw garlic and apply to the boil. It stings but is very effective.

- Eat 3 to 4 cloves of garlic daily while the boil is still active.

- 4 ounces mung beans, $\frac{1}{2}$ ounce kombu, raw brown sugar. Cook together in 4 cups water until reduced to half. Eat throughout the day.

Bowel - bloody

- 4 ounces bean curd, 1 ounce raw brown sugar. Cook together and eat every other day. Cook fresh every day.

Bowel - constipation or sluggish

- Drink fresh pear juice. Plum or mulberry juice make acceptable substitutes.

- Eat popcorn without butter or salt.

- Eat a banana early in the morning.

- Drink a warm glass of water and lemon juice.

- Drink the juice of a raw potato, hot water, and honey.

- Boil and drink 1 ounce crushed black sesame seeds and $\frac{1}{2}$ cup water.

- Eat two apples daily, morning and evening.

Bronchitis - chronic

- 6 ounces chestnuts, 5 ounces pork. Braise together. Eat twice daily.

Chest - tight

- Eat spinach soup.

Corns or warts

- Alternate dropping a drop of castor oil and fresh cranberry juice on the skin several times a day. Cover with a Band-Aid.™

Cough

- Juice 1 pound celery and a pinch of salt. Boil together in an earthenware pot. Drink first thing in the morning and later in the evening.

- Steam 1 pound of papaya. Eat with raw brown sugar 4 times a day.

- At the first onset of the cough, crush one or two cloves of garlic. Pour in 3 to 5 teaspoons of hot water, stir well, and drink all of it. Repeat 2 to 3 times a day. The cough will usually stop within 12 hours or sooner.

Cough - dry

- 4 ounces black sesame seeds, 2 ounces raw brown sugar. Crush together and eat two times a day.

Cough - with phlegm

- 5 ounces fresh trout, 1 fresh tomato, black pepper. Cook together in ¾ cup water for 10 minutes. Drink while lukewarm.

Diarrhea

- First, avoid any cold food, cold drink, raw fruit, fruit juice, or milk. Stay warm.

- Eat crackers and carbonated water every 2 hours until symptoms disapper.

- Toast 6 ounces buckwheat in a dry pan without oil. Grind into a powder, mix with ½ ounces warm water, and drink twice a day.

- Toast 6 ounces brown rice in a dry pan without oil until brown. Add 2 cups of water and cook for 30 minutes. Add a pinch of salt. Eat and drink 4 to 5 times a day.

Diarrhea - chronic

- 4 ounces raw carrot, 2 ounces raw brown sugar. Cook in 3 cups water until reduced to half. Eat and drink all of it.

Eyes - sties or red swollen eyes

- Boil an egg, shell it, then roll on the affected eye while the egg is still warm. Reduces swelling and redness.

- Drop one drop of fresh lemon juice into the eye. Be cautious; this will cause burning sensation in the eyes.

- Drop 2 to 3 drops of a mixture of salt and distilled water into each eye. Do one eye at a time. It will sting very badly, but is very effective.

- Wet 2 bags of herb tea and apply one bag to each eye.

Eyes - tired or poor eyesight due to strain

- Boil ½ teaspoon of fennel seed in water, either alone or with chamomile. Strain and use as an eyewash. Avoid fennel plants that have been sprayed with chemicals.

Fever - high

- 8 ounces distilled water, $\frac{1}{2}$ lemon, honey to taste. Mix and drink 2 to 3 times a day.

- Use vinegar to wash the back and armpits. Put sliced lemon on the forehead and temples.

Flatulence

- Add two teaspoons of cloves to a pint of hot water. Allow to soften for 30 minutes in a covered container. Strain and drink as a tea.

Hiccups

- Make ginger tea with honey. Drink for 10 minutes.

Hemorrhoids

- Eat one orange 3 times a day.

- Eat two bananas early in the morning on an empty stomach.

Hyperacidity

- 8 clams toasted in their shells. Eat twice daily every other day for one week.

Hypertension

- Take 3 tablespoons of rice vinegar or cider with each meal every day.

- 3 ounces crushed sunflower seeds, 6 ounces fresh celery juice. Mix and drink twice daily. Continue for 20 to 30 days.

Impotence - due to kidney deficiency.

- Eat 3 ounces fresh walnuts once a day for 30 days.

- Steam 10 ounces of fresh shrimp. Eat with brandy once a day for 20 days.

- 4 ounces mussels, 4 ounces lean pork, 2 cloves garlic, 2 potatoes, 2 cups water. Boil together for 20 minutes. Eat twice daily for 6 to 12 days.

Laryngitis

- 5 ounces dried figs, 2 ounces molasses, 1 cup water. Boil until reduced to half. Eat and drink twice a day.

Leg weakness

- 5 ounces minced lean beef, 2 slices fresh ginger, $1\frac{1}{2}$ cups water. Boil and drink at night while still hot.

Lymph glands - swollen

- 1 medium raw potato, 1 glass water. Blend, drain, and drink the juice every day for 10 days.

Menstruation

- Dried dates, raw brown sugar, fresh ginger, 2 cups water. Cook for 10 minutes. Eat and drink once a day for 5 days.

Nose bleed - chronic

- 1 pound catfish, few stalks spring onion. Steam and eat every other day for a week.

Parasites

- Eat 2 to 3 ounces raw sunflower seeds daily for 10 days.

Prostate gland - infected

- Eat 2 ounces raw sunflower seeds or pumpkin seeds daily for 10 days.

Seasickness/Airplane Sickness

- Drink ginger tea 1 day prior to travelling.

- Take ginger tablets while travelling.

Snake bite

- Mash raw eggplant and apply to the bite.

Sweating - excessive

- 3 ounces fresh oysters, 1 ounce oyster shells. Boil in 3 cups water until reduced to half. Eat and drink twice daily.

Throat - sore

- 1 ounce spring onion, 1 cup water. Boil for 5 minutes. Drink throughout the day.

- Boil watermelon skin in 2 cups water until reduced to half. Drink 2 to 3 times daily.

Urination - frequent

- 2 ounces fresh walnuts toasted until brown. Warm a glass of rice wine or sake. Eat and drink the two together once or twice a day.

Urination - painful

- Eat a pear or some watermelon.

- Drink the juice of sweet corn or corn silk tea.

Urination - retention

- Eat a fresh carrot.

- 4 ounces mung beans, 2 cups water, raw brown sugar. Cook, eat, and drink while still warm.

Urination - sluggish

- Drink 5 fluid ounces fresh plum juice.

- Drink 6 fluid ounces fresh pear juice before breakfast.

- Cook and eat brown rice.

FOODS DURING ILLNESS OR WEAKNESS

When a person gets sick, the immune system is weakened. The body becomes vulnerable, as it has temporarily lost its source of resistance against outside invaders. For this reason, special attention to diet is required until the body can regain its defenses. If you know how to take care of yourself, you can recover from an oncoming illness in 24 hours or less. If you eat the wrong foods at the wrong time, however, they may exacerbate the condition and you may be dragging around for weeks or months. Eating certain foods at these critical times can actually help avert an oncoming illness. I you're feeling weak, you can have a dramatic effect on your own health and vitality by following a few dietary rules. Here are some basic practices to follow when you or somebody you care for has become ill.

PROTECTION WHEN THE BODY HAS LOW ENERGY

Someone who has no energy or low energy must protect body surfaces from exposure in order to help the body conserve strength. A person in this condition should not take a long shower or bath until they are feeling stronger, especially if they have a runny nose. Taking long showers can weaken the energy surrounding the body. A quick shower is all right. If a person is really weak or shaking, try to minimize exposing their skin to the air and to running water. To cleanse them, wipe them off with a damp cloth using warm water and cover them quickly afterwards.

Mental concentration can also drain the energy of weak people. For this reason, they should not watch TV or read a book until they are stronger. TV also exposes the body to radiation which can weaken the immune system.

COMBATTING A FEVER

If a person is feverish, don't cover them up too much because it will increase their temperature. At the same time, don't let them expose themselves too much either. Have them wear light, long-sleeved clothes and pants. Drafts and windy places should be avoided.

Sometimes fevers are caused by constipation. Toxins from the liver may not have been eliminated daily, and their back-up into the blood stream will create heat in the body. This condition can be counteracted by eating foods which help eliminate toxins through the urine or feces, such as barley soup with okra, chamomile tea, or corn silk tea. (See the home remedy section for recipes to relieve a high fever.)

FOODS TO AVOID AND TO EAT DURING WEAKNESS OR FEVER

Fried foods and raw food should not be eaten by a person feeling weak or with a fever. Fried foods increase body temperature, exacerbating a fever. Raw food requires a lot of energy to digest inside the body. This energy should rather be conserved for rebuilding strength. Use the energy of your stove to cook food so that your patient's energy will not be further depleted. Other foods that should be avoided because they require a lot of energy to digest are acid roots, fruit juice, and mung beans. Barley soup, chicken broth, vegetable soup, bean thread soup, and ginger tea are very helpful in rebuilding strength in the body's energy.

REST

Rest is, of course, the foremost contributor to fast recuperation. You should never underestimate its value. If you die tomorrow, the world will still continue to rotate and everyone will continue to go about their daily routines without you. So don't worry that you need to get back to work right away. It can wait for you. Take the time to rest so your body will regain its resiliency.

CONGEE

Congee is widely used in Vietnam and many East Asian countries to nurture a weak person back to strength. Growing up, I remember eating congee whenever I showed signs of oncoming illness. It is traditionally used to strengthen the digestive system since it is very easy to digest. For this reason it is an excellent breakfast for the elderly and can be eaten daily. With different herbs, seeds, or nuts, it can be effective in strengthening the immune system or increasing circulation. For example, the following herbs with congee will have different effects upon the body's energy system:

- Ginger promotes Qi, blood, and warms the middle burner.

- Honey nourishes the heart, calms the spirit, and lubricates the intestines.

- Walnuts tonify the kidney yang and nourish the brain.

- Chestnuts tonify the kidney yin and strengthen the Jing.

The following is a basic recipe for congee that is good for a cold or the flu.

CONGEE RECIPE

1 cup of rice
6 cups of water

(1)
Chopped pork, mung beans, or barley
Chopped peeled shrimp

(2)
Spring onions cut finely
Ginger (thumb-size) chopped finely
Black pepper
Fish sauce to taste (or miso or tamari)

Start with one of the items in group (1). Pork makes a good choice because it lowers liver heat. This heat could eventually cause a sore throat or headache since the liver meridian travels through the throat to the eyes, and to the top of the head. If you don't like pork or you are a vegetarian, you may want to use mung beans, which help to cool a fever-ish condition. If you are anemic, then use barley.

Place rice and water in a heavy-lidded pot. If you are cooking with mung beans, start them with the rice. Cook for about two hours on medium heat. Stir once in awhile to prevent burning on the bottom. When the rice is cooked and is soft like porridge, add ingredients from (1) and (2). Cook for 15 minutes if cooking with pork. Cook for 5 minutes if cooking with shrimp. Serve warm. This soup will make you perspire and urinate often. This will promote circulation and help the body eliminate toxic wastes.

The congee can be reheated during the day if you or your patient is very sick or weak. It should be eaten four to five times a day. Never serve leftovers from the day before. It should be prepared fresh every day. As shown below, different ingredients added to congee will help in treating different symptom patterns and conditions.

CONDITION	INGREDIENT TO ADD TO CONGEE
Dampness in the spleen. Sluggish feeling due to muscle soreness. Edema. Gout. Excessive urine retention. Dysuria (difficult urination). Other kidney and bladder problems.	Adzuki Bean
Need to harmonize and moisten the viscera.	Spinach
Liver yang ascension. Top headache due to anger or emotional upsets.	Celery
Chronic diarrhea.	Leek
Diabetes. Jaundice.	Water Chestnut
Weak kidneys. Lower back and knee pain and weakness. Anal hemorrhages.	Chestnut

FOODS TO AVOID UNDER CERTAIN CONDITIONS

As stated earlier, the timely application of an appropriate diet can avert oncoming illness. Conversely, eating the wrong foods at the wrong time can exacerbate a developing condition and further weaken the immune system, causing additional delays in healing time. In fact, it may be that you need to immediately delete an item from your diet that you have been consuming on a regular basis.

Certain ailments are more sensitive than others to food intake. The next table highlights some common ailments which can be adversely affected by the foods described. These food should be carefully avoided when the body is experiencing the associated conditions.

CONDITION	FOODS TO AVOID
Boils.	Chicken meat, shrimp, crab, fish.
Colds/flu with runny nose or congestion.	Chicken, goose, duck, pork, rice. Chicken is the worst because it increases coughing, stuffy nose, and congestion problems.
Heart disease.	Alcohol, spicy foods, deep fried foods.
Hypertension.	Bok choy, fried foods, roasted food, nuts, alcohol, coffee, tea containing caffeine, tobacco, salt. Decrease meat consumption.
Lung problems / asthma / bronchitis.	Sour, spicy, cold, fatty, deep fried foods. Daikon, tobacco, alcohol.
Stomach / intestinal problems.	Steak, roast beef, eggs, cake, sweet rice, sweet potatoes, daikon, sour foods, fruits, cold and leftover foods.
Emotional pain from indulging in anger.	Sour, cold, leftover foods. Coffee.
Skin eruptions and disease.	Spicy foods.
Ulcers and /or pus.	Peanuts, yellow beans, eggs, sesame seeds.

recipes for health

Cooking for Nourishment and Nurture

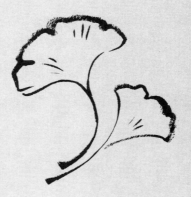

PREPARING FOOD FOR BODY, MIND, AND SPIRIT

*i*n the recipes in this section, it is not my intent to give you an exhaustive list of recipes but rather to share some basic ones that will help to make your cooking easier and more enjoyable. I want to encourage you to add and subtract ingredients to suit your taste or health condition. For instance, the amounts of water listed in some of the recipes for soups can be varied depending on whether you want a thinner soup or one with more of a stew consistency. You will have to use your intuition in these cases. Some recipes won't be for you. Blackened Grouper, for instance, raises body heat and dries out body fluids and should not be eaten by those experiencing constipation.

Remember to cook with consciousness and love in order to receive the greatest benefit from the food you prepare. Integrate the knowledge you have gained from reading with the intuition that flows from within yourself. Create a meal and pay attention to how it makes you feel. Make adjustments as you experiment. Your food should suit your feelings for the day. In this way, the ongoing process of nurturing your health and spiritual development will never become stagnant. Enjoy!

BEVERAGES

GINGER TEA

Cut a thumb-sized piece of ginger. Peel the skin off and cut the ginger into thin slices. Boil 4 cups of water, then add ginger. Turn to low heat for 10 minutes. Drink the tea 3–4 times daily. Add maple syrup, honey, or blackstrap molasses to sweeten.

NUT MILK

1 cup raw cashews of almonds
3½–4 cups water
2–6 dates (optional)
¼ tsp. salt

Mix nuts, salt, dates and 1–2 cups water in a blender until the mixture forms a smooth liquid paste. Then add 2 more cups of water and blend again. If desired, you can substitute banana or other fruit for flavor/sweetness instead of the dates. Use over cereals. Also useful for sweetening or sauces in cooking.

GREEN COCKTAIL

1 qt. of fresh carrot juice
8 oz. of wheat grass juice
1 stalk of celery
several springs of parsley
1 fresh tomato
kelp to taste

Mix all ingredients in a blender. Drink in moderation to promote Qi.

NUTRITION DRINK

1 fertile egg yolk
8 oz. Perrier water
½ fresh lemon or lime juice
honey to taste

Mix all ingredients briefly in a blender or with a whisk.

A revitalizing drink for those who are sick and weak. This is an old formula that is also used in some oriental countries to nourish the body after having sex.

OAT DRINK

5 oz. distilled water
½ cup rolled oats
½ tsp. of honey or pure maple syrup
Tahini or almond, peanut or cashew butter

Mix all ingredients in a blender and drink for breakfast.

DRESSINGS AND SAUCES

ARTICHOKE DIP

1 tbsp. mayonnaise
½ tsp. horseradish
1 tbsp. ketchup
1 squeeze of lime juice

Mix all ingredients together and serve with fresh steamed artichokes.

GREEN SALAD DRESSING

2 tbsp. lemon juice
1 cucumber, thinly peeled
1 green onion with tops
$\frac{1}{2}$ cup cashews
1 tsp. onion salt

Mix all ingredients in a blender. Wonderful as a salad dressing or dip.

GUACAMOLE SPREAD OR DRESSING

2 ripe avocados
1 tbsp. lemon juice
$\frac{1}{2}$ tsp. salt
Trace garlic salt
1 hearty slice fresh tomato (may use canned tomatoes)
2 tsp. onion, chopped

Mash avocados with a whisk or in a blender until smooth. Add salt, garlic salt, and lemon juice. Chop tomato and onion finely and combine all ingredients. Chill covered to keep avocados from turning dark. You can make a salad dressing consistency by adding a small amount of water.

HOMEMADE VINAIGRETTE SALAD DRESSING

2 tbsp. soy sauce
1 tsp. raw sugar
1 tbsp. vinegar
1 tbsp. olive oil

Pinch of oregano
Pinch of thyme
A few slices of onion

Mix all ingredients and toss with Boston lettuce

CASHEW GRAVY

2 cups hot water
½ cup cashews
½ tsp. salt
2 tsp. onion powder
2 tbsp. corn starch or arrowroot

Mix ingredients in a blender until smooth. Pour into a small saucepan and bring to a boil. Use as a white sauce. Add 2 tbsp. of food yeast for gravy.

GOLDEN SAUCE

1 small potato
½ small carrot
1⅓ cups of water
2 tbsp. cashews
¾ tsp. salt
2 tbsp. fresh lemon juice
Dash celery salt

Cook potato, carrot, and water together in a small saucepan. When done, blend with other ingredients. Serve over broccoli, cauliflower, or other vegetables.

NUOC MAM SAUCE (FISH SAUCE)

Fresh chili pepper, seeded
1 clove garlic, peeled
1 tsp. raw sugar
½ medium lime
1 tsp. vinegar
1 tbsp. water
4 tbsp. fish sauce
Mortar and pestle

Crush the pepper and garlic together in the mortar with the sugar. If you are not sure how hot you want your sauce, start with a small amount of pepper. Add more later if desired. Peel and seed the lime and squeeze the pulp into the mortar with the garlic and pepper. Add vinegar and water to the pulp mixture and mix well. Add the fish sauce (plain nuoc mam) last. Can be stored in the refrigerator for up to 2–3 months in a tightly closed bottle or jar.

QUICK AND EASY GRAVY

⅓ cup whole grain flour
½ tsp. onion powder
1 tsp. chicken seasoning or another of your favorites.

Tumble ingredients in a dry skillet until slightly browned. Stir in water until you achieve a desired thickness and simmer for a few minutes.

SOY SAUCE MIXTURE

2 tbsp. soy sauce
1 tbsp. raw sugar

1 tbsp. water
Chopped garlic (optional)
Chopped red hot chili (optional)
One squeeze of a lemon

Mix together and use as a condiment.

Lemon can be added to counteract the taste of soy sauce when you feel that it is an overriding taste in this recipe or any other.

TARTAR SAUCE

1 tbsp. each chopped onion,
  green pepper, parsley, cucumber,
  and olives
Salt, paprika, and dill weed to taste

Mix the above ingredients with 1 cup of tofu mayonnaise. (See recipe under *Spreads and Condiments*.) Let stand overnight in the refrigerator.

SPREADS & CONDIMENTS

BEAN SPREAD

1 cup well-cooked beans
$\frac{1}{8}$ tsp. sweet basil
Dash garlic powder
$\frac{1}{2}$ tsp. onion salt
Salt to taste

Blend beans with enough bean juice or water to enable blender to turn. For gravy, just add more water. Mix in seasonings.

GAMISIO

15 parts sesame seeds
1 part sea salt

Heat a skillet using medium to low heat. Using no oil, roast sea salt and sesame seeds, stirring frequently until light brown. When cool, crush mixture with a pestle and put in a jar. Keep refrigerated. Use on rice or salad.

HERBAL SALT

Garlic
Dill
Onion
Nettles
Basil
Marjoram
Papaya leaves
Celery seed
Comfrey leaves
Kelp powder

Blend the above herbs to taste. Kelp powder should make up one third of the total mixture.

TOFU MAYONNAISE

1 tsp. onion salt
¼ tsp. garlic salt
2 tsp. fresh lemon juice
2 cups tofu
¾ cup water

Blend until smooth.

SOUPS AND STEWS

BARLEY SOUP

1 16-oz. can of barley
½ gallon water
¼ cup adzuki beans
½ cup carrots, cut into ¼" squares
1 cup broccoli, cut into bite-sized pieces

Soak adzuki beans in hot water for about 2 hours to avoid gas after eating. Add fresh water and cook overnight in a slow cooker. The next day, add barley, carrots, and broccoli and cook for another ½ hour on medium heat. Season with rosemary, thyme, and shoyu to taste. This is a very nutritious soup for vegetarians.

BLACK BEAN SOUP

½ lb. black beans, rinsed and soaked overnight
1 medium onion, chopped
1 bay leaf
A pinch of pepper
2 tomatoes, peeled and chopped
½ gal. of water
2 cloves garlic, chopped
1 tsp. oregano
1 tbsp. olive oil
2 tsp. parsley, chopped

Place all ingredients in a large pot. Cook for 2 hours over medium-low heat. Serve with rice.

This recipe may be cooked in a slow cooker overnight or before leaving for work so that you will have fresh soup waiting for you when you come home from work.

CHICKEN SOUP OR CHICKEN BROTH

1 chicken, cut into 4 sections
1 gallon of water
1 onion
1 thumb-sized piece of ginger
Fish sauce to taste

Clean chicken well—inside and out, after cutting into 4 sections. Boil 1 gallon of water with onion, ginger, and fish sauce. Add chicken sections and continue to cook at a low rolling boil. When cooked, bone the chicken and put the meat back into the broth. Simmer in a slow cooker overnight (about 8 hours) or start cooking before going to work in the morning. Later, divide the broth into small jars and keep in the refrigerator for use throughout the week.

When you come home from work each day, start a pot of rice cooking. Warm one of the jars of chicken broth and add vegetables like carrots, potatoes, green beans, and peas for making vegetable soup. Or you can use this chicken / vegetable broth as a soup base for making squash or butternut soup. Watercress or cabbage can be added to the other vegetables, or you can add ABC noodles for ABC soup.

FISH STEW

1 lb. trout or any white meat fish
2 tomatoes cut into 6 pieces
2 stalks sliced celery
1 green onion cut finely
6 cups water
Fish sauce or tamari sauce
Some black pepper to taste

Boil the water and add tamari or fish sauce. Bring to a boil again and add celery, tomato, fish, and green onion. Adjust pepper to taste. Serve with rice.

GINGER TOFU SOUP

2 pieces of tofu cut into 1-inch squares
½ lb. spinach washed and cut into 2-inch long pieces
2 tsp. miso
3 slices of ginger
5 cups of water
Soy sauce to taste
Black pepper to taste

Bring water to a boil and add the miso, tofu, and ginger. Bring to a boil again and add the spinach. Cook briefly. (Remember that fresh spinach doesn't need to cook long.) Sprinkle in black pepper as desired. Serve with brown rice and steamed spring onions.

MAGNIFICENT MINESTRONE

1 cup cooked garbanzo beans (¼ cup dried)
1 cup cooked navy beans (¼ cup dried)
1 cup cooked kidney beans (¼ cup dried)
1½ qts. water or vegetable stock
½ cup barley
2 stalks celery, chopped
1 carrot, thinly sliced
Salt to taste
1 12-oz. can tomato juice
2 tbsp. olive oil

1 onion, chopped
½ cup parsley, chopped
½ cup spinach, chopped
2 cloves garlic, smashed
1 tsp. oregano
1 bay leaf
1 tbsp. tamari sauce
1 16-oz. can whole peeled tomatoes, chopped

Soak beans overnight. Cook until tender in water. Add barley, celery, carrots, and tomatoes. Sauté onion, parsley, spinach, garlic, and herbs in olive oil until tender. Add these to the soup. Simmer while covered for 1 hour.

MILLET SOUP

½ cup millet
¼ cup barley
½ cup lentils
½ gallon water
Soy sauce or herbal salt to taste

Cook all ingredients for 3 to 4 hours on low heat. Add herbal salt to taste. You can eat this for breakfast or as a snack.

MISO SOUP

1 4″ strip of nori, soaked and sliced
½ cup tofu, cut into ½″ squares
1 pint of water
2 tbsp. pureed miso
2 tbsp. green onion, chopped
Shoyu to taste

Boil nori in water and add tofu. Cook until tofu and nori are soft. Turn heat to simmer and add miso. Stir miso well, dissolving it into the soup. Simmer for 2–3 minutes. Add the green onion last. Season with shoyu to taste.

This is a basic miso soup. You can add vegetables, such as carrots, peas or mushrooms. Or you can use a different seaweed for a different flavor. If you add watercress or some other tender vegetable, do not overcook. Use your own judgment as to the quantity of ingredients to use.

NAVY BEAN SOUP

$\frac{1}{2}$ lbs. navy beans
1 tbsp. olive oil
$\frac{1}{2}$ tsp. cumin powder
1 medium onion, chopped
2 tbsp. sweet miso
Soy sauce to taste

Soak navy beans overnight or for one hour in hot water. Discard the water. Boil one pint of fresh water and add miso and navy beans. Cook on medium heat for one hour.

In a skillet, heat oil and add chopped onion and cumin powder. Cook until mixture turns light brown. Add skillet mixture to the soup. Add soy sauce to taste. Serve with crackers or rice.

NORI SOUP

$\frac{1}{2}$ tsp. sesame oil
$\frac{1}{2}$ medium onion sliced
3 oz. fresh mushrooms
2 pints water

2 sheets of nori
5 tbsp. of shoyu
1 spring onion chopped to garnish

Brush a deep pot with sesame oil and heat. Add the onion and a few drops of shoyu. Sauté until fragrant. Add mushrooms and sauté for 2 to 3 more minutes. Add water and bring to a boil. Break the nori sheet into small pieces and add to the soup. Simmer for 5 minutes. Add the shoyu and stir. Garnish with a green onion.

SHRIMP AND BEAN THREAD SOUP

½ lb. shelled shrimp
3 cups of water
1 tbsp. fish sauce
1 green onion, sliced thin
1 4-oz. pkg. of bean thread

Cover bean thread in warm water and soak for about 10 minutes or until soft. Cut into pieces about 2 to 3 inches long. Bring water to a boil in a soup pot on high heat and add the fish sauce. Drop the shrimp into the boiling water. Add bean thread and let boil for one minute. Stir, cover, and cook for 3 minutes on medium heat. Turn heat off. Sprinkle the surface with green onion and black pepper.

TURKEY SOUP

2 turkey drumsticks
2 medium carrots, cut into bite-sized pieces
1 stalk celery, cut into ⅓″ pieces
1 thumb-sized piece of ginger
2 bay leaves

2 pints of water
4 medium potatoes, cut into bite-sized pieces
2 fresh tomatoes, cut into small pieces
1 medium onion, peeled
Salt to taste

Bring water to a boil. Add turkey drumsticks, onion, and ginger. Cook for ½ hour. Add carrots, potatoes, celery, tomatoes and ginger. Cook for another ½ hour over medium heat. Add salt or soy sauce to taste. You may bone the drumsticks before serving if desired. Serve with rice.

This recipe may be cooked in a slow cooker overnight so that you can have a fresh soup for breakfast, lunch, and dinner.

VEGETARIAN SOUP

3 potatoes with skins, cut into bite-sized pieces
½ cup garbanzo beans, soaked overnight
1 leek, cut into 1″ pieces
½ tsp. sea salt
1 large tomato
10 cups of water
1 onion, chopped
1 chayote, cut into bite-sized pieces.

Bring water to a boil. Add potatoes, garbanzos, tomato, chayote, and onion. Bring to a boil again. Then turn heat down to low and cook for one hour. Add leeks and bring to a boil again. Cook briefly. Serve with rice.

If you do not like garbanzo beans, substitute black beans, kidney beans, adzuki beans, or lentils.

WHOLE GRAINS & LEGUMES

ADZUKI BEAN RICE

1 cup brown rice
1 cup adzuki beans
1 piece of kombu 3"–6" long
4 cups water
Salt to taste

Wash adzuki beans. Boil 2 cups of water with the beans and kombu for 20 minutes. Cool the beans until lukewarm. Wash rice. Put rice, adzuki beans, broth and kombu into a pressure cooker. Cook together for 25 minutes. Add salt to taste.

BROWN RICE

1 cup rice
3 cups water

Put rice in a pot and add water. Cover pot and place on high heat until it boils. Watch carefully to be sure it doesn't boil over. Cook covered over high heat for 10 minutes or until the water and rice come to the same level. Turn heat to low. Let simmer for 20–30 minutes.

HOMEMADE BREAD

5 cups water
½ cup dates
1 cup oats
1½ tbsp. lecithin granules
1 tbsp. salt
½ cup gluten flour

3 tbsp. yeast
5 cups whole grain flour
Raisins, walnuts, sunflower seeds, or onions

Blend the water and dates until smooth. Pour into a large bowl and add the remaining ingredients. Beat this vigorously for a count of 100. Then add about 4 more cups of flour, one at a time. Knead 10 minutes. The more you knead, the better the texture. Divide the dough into 4 loaves and put into well oiled bread pans. Let rise in preheated oven at 140°F until the dough has doubled in size. Then raise the heat to 325°F and bake 35 minutes. Remove from pans and let cool on racks. Raisins, walnuts, sunflower seeds, onion, or other flavorful ingredients can be added to the dough to vary the flavor.

KICHEREE

½ cup mung beans or lentils
½ cup brown rice
1 tsp. ground coriander
⅓ tsp. turmeric
2 tbsp. sesame oil
Pinch of cumin seed
4 cups water

Mix mung beans or lentils with brown rice and sauté in sesame oil with coriander, turmeric, and cumin seed. Add water and simmer for 20–25 minutes.

LENTIL-NUT LOAF

1 cup cooked lentils (red or green)
¼ cup whole rye flour

½ cup wheat germ
½ cup tomato sauce
1 tbsp. nutritional yeast (optional)
1 tbsp. tamari sauce
2 cups ground nuts (walnuts, pecans, or almonds)

Combine the above ingredients in a bowl.

Sauté the following in a pan:
¼ cup vegetable oil
1 onion, chopped
¼ cup parsley, chopped
4 mushrooms, chopped
1 10-oz. bag fresh spinach, chopped
1 clove garlic, mashed
1 tsp. oregano

Combine all ingredients together in the bowl. Shape into a loaf, and bake in a loaf pan at 350°F for 30 minutes. Serve with any tomato sauce, olives, or mushroom gravy.

SESAME RICE

2 cups rice
½ cup roasted white or black sesame seeds
4½ cups water

Wash sesame seeds quickly. Combine ingredients and cook as you would usually cook your rice.

SWEET RICE

2½ cups of water
2 cups sweet rice

1 tbsp. sesame seeds
Kombu (optional)

Bring water to a boil and add rice. When water begins to boil again, stir slowly until it becomes heavy and rice and water come to the same level. Lower the heat and cover with a lid. Cook for 5–7 minutes longer. Add sesame seeds. Stir again. 3 minutes later, turn the heat off.

You may add kombu after soaking it for 10 minutes. Put it in the rice when you are ready to turn the heat to low.

MEAT DISHES

CHICKEN BREAST AND BROCCOLI

2 lbs. chicken
2 lbs. steamed broccoli
2 tbsp. soy sauce
2 tsp. rice wine or cooking wine
$3\frac{1}{2}$ tbsp. water
3 tsp. cornstarch
1 tbsp. green onion, chopped
1 tbsp. ginger root, chopped
1 tbsp. garlic, chopped
1 tsp. raw sugar
$\frac{1}{2}$ tsp. sesame oil
$\frac{1}{3}$ tsp. Szechuan peppercorn powder

Cut chicken into $1\frac{1}{2}''$ long matchstick pieces. Mix 1 tbsp. soy sauce, 1 tsp. wine, 2 tbsp. water, and 2 tbsp. cornstarch in a bowl. Stir chicken into the mixture and then let soak for 20 minutes. Heat $\frac{1}{4}$ tsp. sesame oil to medium heat in a pan. Add onion, ginger root, and garlic and stir-fry until fragrant. Add chicken pieces to stir-fry with 1 tsp. wine, 1 tbsp. soy sauce, 1 tsp. raw sugar, $\frac{1}{4}$ tsp. sesame oil, $1\frac{1}{2}$ tbsp. water, 1 tsp. cornstarch and peppercorn powder. Continue to stir-fry and mix. Remove to a serving plate. Position pre-steamed broccoli on both sides of chicken and serve with rice.

NOTE: Use grain-fed chicken for all recipes requiring chicken.

CHICKEN CHILI

3 tbsp. safflower oil
1 large onion, chopped
4 chicken breast halves, skinned, boned, and cubed.
2 cloves garlic, minced fine
4 cups sliced stewed tomatoes
1 small sweet red pepper, chopped
1 jalapeno pepper, minced
4 oz. pitted black olives
2 tbsp. whole cumin seeds, toasted
¼ tsp. ground cinnamon
¼ tsp. crushed dried red chilies
2 tbsp. oregano
2 cups water or 1 cup dark beer

Heat oil in a large skillet. Brown chicken with onion and garlic for 10 minutes. Add the rest of the ingredients. Cook for 30 minutes.

If you are a vegetarian, replace chicken with 2 cups of dried kidney beans.

CHICKEN WITH GINGER

1 lb. chicken, cleaned well and cut into bite-sized pieces.
1 thumb-sized piece of ginger, cut into toothpick pieces
1 clove garlic, chopped fine

3 tsp. fish sauce
1 tsp. cooking oil

Sauté garlic and ginger in a heated skillet with oil until fragrant. Stir in fish sauce and add chicken. Cover with a lid for 5-7 minutes. Serve with brown rice and green vegetables.

CHICKEN SALAD

4 chicken thighs
1 lb. white cabbage, cut into ⅛″ slices
2 quarts of water
5 tbsp. sea salt
1 tbsp. tamari or soy sauce
¼ cup chopped roasted peanuts
1 cup vinegar
2 tbsp. safflower oil
3 tbsp. raw brown sugar
⅛ tsp. black pepper
1 medium onion, chopped fine
Fresh bay leaves or cilantro, cut fine

Boil chicken thighs in lightly salted water for 10 minutes. Remove chicken and let cool. Store broth for soup recipes. Bone and skin chicken when it cools. Soak sliced cabbage in a mixture of 2 quarts of water and 5 tbsp. of sea salt for 15 minutes. Rinse and squeeze out excess water. Place in a big stainless steel bowl. Pour in a mixture of tamari, vinegar, safflower oil, raw brown sugar, black pepper, and onion. Add chicken meat, mix well, and place on a plate. Garnish with peanuts and fresh bay leaves.

BLACKENED GROUPER

1 lb. grouper
¼ tsp. black pepper
¼ tsp. white pepper
¼ tsp. cayenne pepper

Mix together peppers on a plate. Dip grouper in soy sauce and then roll in the pepper mixture. Fry in a skillet with cooking oil for about 5 minutes. Increase or decrease pepper for spicier or milder grouper. Serve with rice and potatoes and steamed kale, steamed collard greens, or steamed okra.

BROILED FLOUNDER

1 lb. flounder
2 tbsp. mayonnaise
Salt and pepper to taste
1 egg white
½ medium onion, chopped fine
Pinch of rosemary (optional)

Mix together egg white, mayonnaise, onion, salt, pepper, and rosemary. Spread mixture over flounder. Broil until fish is opaque and flakes easily. Eat with rice and steamed broccoli or steamed asparagus.

SEA TROUT WITH FRESH TOMATOES

1 medium sea trout, cleaned well
3 ripe tomatoes, chopped fine
½ onion, sliced
Pinch of black pepper

2 tbsp. soy sauce
Spinach, washed thoroughly and steamed slightly
   (or substitute with watercress)
1 tsp. cooking oil
1 clove garlic, chopped fine
1 cup of distilled water

Pour oil into a skillet on medium heat. Add onion and garlic. Sauté until fragrant. Add fish, chopped tomatoes, and soy sauce. Cook for 10 minutes. In another pan, steam spinach and set on a dish. Place fish in the center and pour the juice of the fish over top. Sprinkle with black pepper. Serve with rice.

GRILLED SHRIMP

1 lb. shrimp with shell
½ cup fresh pineapple juice
1 tbsp. soy sauce

Marinate shrimp in a mixture of the pineapple juice and soy sauce for a few seconds. Grill and serve with a baked potato, steamed broccoli, or zucchini.

SHRIMP WITH PINEAPPLE

½ lb. medium shrimp
2 green onions
¼ fresh pineapple
1 tbsp. safflower oil
2 tbsp. fish sauce
Dash of black pepper of fresh mint

Shell the shrimp, wash them well, and chop coarsely. Chop the onion finely and mix with the shrimp. Chop the fresh pineapple into small chunks. Heat the oil in a skillet and sauté the shrimp with the onion for about one minute. Add pineapple and cook for 2 minutes. Add fish sauce. Remove the mixture and place on a plate. Garnish with fresh mint. Serve with warm rice.

To vary recipe, you may want to replace pineapple with turnips, okra, or any other vegetable of your choice.

SPRING ROLLS

Rice paper
Rice noodles
Shrimp, unshelled
Fresh herbs of your choice
Bean Sprouts
Bean paste
Chopped garlic
Salt

Wash shrimp in a mixture of 1 tsp. salt and 1 pint water. Bring fresh water to a boil, add shrimp. Bring to a boil again, just long enough to cook shrimp without causing them to shrink and become chewy. Set aside in a colander to drain and shell when cool. Shelling after cooking preserves nutrients and makes shrimp tastier.

Bring another pot of water to a boil. Add rice noodles and bring to a boil again for 2–3 minutes. Drain noodles in a colander.

Wash bean sprouts. Sauté chopped garlic in 1 tsp. cooking oil. Mix in 5 tsp. bean paste. Place shrimp, herbs, rice noodles, and sprouts on wet rice paper. Fold like an egg roll. Serve with bean paste sauce.

STIR-FRIED SEAFOOD AND VEGETABLES

½ lb. scallops, cleaned
1 lb. shrimp, shelled, deveined and ends cut off
¼ lb. sweet peas
½ lb. baby corn
2 tsp. oyster sauce
6–8 black mushrooms, soaked and stems cut off
8 oz. water chestnuts, washed
2 tsp. cooking oil
2 cloves garlic, chopped fine
Pinch of coriander

Heat frying pan with 1 tsp. oil and ½ of garlic until fragrant. Add scallops, shrimp, and 1 tsp. oyster sauce. Stir for 2 minutes and set aside in a dish. Heat the pan again with 1 tsp. oil and the remainder of the garlic. Add the sweet peas, baby corn, black mushrooms, water chestnuts, and 1 tsp. oyster sauce. Stir for 3 minutes of until slightly done. Combine with scallops and shrimp. Mix together and place on a plate. Sprinkle coriander on top. Serve with brown rice.

PORK CHOPS AND LEMON GRASS

6 pork chops
1 stalk lemon grass, chopped fine
1 clove garlic, chopped fine
3 tsp. soy sauce
1 tsp. cooking oil

Heat a skillet with cooking oil and sauté garlic and lemon grass. Add pork chops and soy sauce. Cover with lid and lower heat to medium. Simmer for 15 minutes. Serve with brown rice and green vegetables.

PORK WITH DAIKON

½ lb. pork or 1 lb. pork rib, cut into bite-sized pieces
3 tbsp. soy sauce or fish sauce
1 tbsp. sesame oil
1 tbsp. raw sugar
1 daikon, cut into 1″ long strips

Heat oil in a skillet, and then add pork, soy sauce, and raw sugar. Cook 5 to 8 minutes. Keep stirring. Add ½ cup of fresh water and daikon. Cook for 20 minutes with skillet covered. Serve over rice with a bowl of soup.

VEGETARIAN DISHES

ARAME WITH SWEET CORN

1 oz. dried arame
1 tbsp. dark sesame oil
1 cup onions, sliced in half
Water
2–3 tbsp. shoyu
2 cups fresh sweet corn kernels

Clean arame and put in a strainer to drain. Oil a frying pan and heat it. Sauté onions for 1–2 minutes, stirring to insure even cooking. Add arame on top and enough water to just cover the onions. Add a little shoyu. Cover and bring to a boil. Then turn flame to medium-low, and simmer for about 20 minutes. Add corn and a little more shoyu to taste. Simmer 10–15 minutes and mix until liquid evaporates.

BAKED BUTTERNUT SQUASH

3 cups butternut squash, cut into large chunks
1 strip kombu, 6″ long
2–3 tbsp. kuzu
2 cups water
Shoyu to taste

Put squash in a baking dish. Add a couple of teaspoons of water to keep it moist while baking. Cover the baking dish and bake in a preheated 350°F oven for 35–40 minutes, or until almost done. Pour water into a pot and add the kombu. Bring to a boil. Then reduce heat to low, cover and simmer for about 15 minutes. Reduce heat to very low. Remove kombu from the pot and set aside for future use. Dilute kuzu in a little cold water and stir into the water with onions. Bring to a boil, stirring constantly to avoid lumping. Reduce heat to low and season lightly with shoyu. Simmer for about 5 minutes. Pour hot kuzu sauce over the baked squash, cover, and bake for several minutes longer.

BAKED VEGETABLES

3 ripe tomatoes
3 yellow zucchini
2 small eggplant
2 tbsp. olive oil
2 tbsp. marjoram and thyme leaves
2 large cloves garlic, sliced thin
1 lemon wedge, sliced thin
1 tbsp. capers
Pinch of salt

Wash all vegetables thoroughly. Slice eggplant and zucchini diagonally into ¼″ pieces. Tomatoes can be halved first and then sliced straight across. Brush 1 tsp. of oil into a baking dish and place all vegetables in the dish. Cover with half the garlic slices, half the marjoram and thyme leaves, and a pinch of salt. Cover dish and bake in the oven at 350°F for 25 minutes or until the vegetables are cooked and juicy. Add the rest of the lemon and herbs. Cook another 7–10 minutes. If the vegetables are too juicy, pour the juice off and set vegetables aside. Then cook the juice down until it reduces to a syrupy sauce. Pour this sauce back on top of the vegetables.

BEAN SALAD

2 hard-boiled eggs, peeled and quartered
½ lb. green beans, trimmed
½ lb. yellow wax beans, trimmed
½ lb. small redskin potatoes, scrubbed
1 tbsp. honey
1 tbsp. hot water
1 tbsp. cider vinegar
1 tbsp. olive oil
1 tbsp. tamari or soy sauce
1 tsp. Dijon mustard
¼ cup onion, chopped
1 tbsp. fresh mint, chopped

Blanch the green and yellow beans in a large pot for 2 minutes or until they cook through but are still crunchy. Plunge into cold water to stop the cooking process, drain, and set aside. Boil potatoes with the skin on and cut potatoes into eighths. Combine beans, potatoes, and eggs and set aside. Heat oil in a skillet and sauté onion until fragrant. Add a mixture of the honey, hot water, cider vinegar, olive oil, tamari, and Dijon mustard to the skillet. Pour all of this on top of the mixture of beans, potatoes, and eggs. Garnish with chopped mint.

BRAISED CHINESE MUSHROOMS AND TOFU

2 lbs. tofu, cut into ½″ squares
3 pre-softened Chinese black mushrooms, cut in half
2 tbsp. safflower oil
¾ cup of soup stock
1 tbsp. soy sauce
1 tsp. cornstarch
2 tsp. water
1 tsp. sesame oil

Heat 2 tbsp. of safflower oil in a skillet and stir-fry mushrooms until fragrant. Add soup stock, soy sauce, and tofu slices. Cover and cook 5 minutes over low heat until the sauce decreases by half. Add cornstarch, water, and sesame oil to thicken sauce. Toss ingredients lightly and remove to serving plate.

COUSCOUS SALAD

2 tbsp. olive oil
1½ tbsp. lemon juice
1 tsp. dried basil
1 tbsp. raw sugar
1 tbsp. tamari
1 cup tofu, cut into bite-sized pieces
1 tbsp. cooking oil
1 clove garlic, minced
½ tsp. cumin
¼ tsp. each of minced fresh ginger, cinnamon, chili powder,
    turmeric, and a pinch of cayenne mixed together
1 cup of water
Pinch of salt
½ cup couscous

½ cup cooked chickpeas
¼ cup raisins

Mix together first six ingredients. Marinate for 10 minutes. Heat oil in a saucepan and add garlic, cumin, and other herb mixture. Stir for 1 minute. Add water and salt and bring to a boil. Gradually stir in couscous in a steady stream. Turn off heat, cover, and let sit for 10 minutes. Gently scrape couscous onto a baking sheet. When cool, break up any lumps with your hands. Stir into the tofu mixture. Add chickpeas and raisins.

GINGER TOFU

1 lb. tofu, cut into ½" squares
¼ cup tamari
1 tbsp. fresh ginger root, minced
½ tsp. raw sugar or honey
½ tsp. ginger
1 tsp. lemon or lime juice
2 tbsp. safflower oil

Marinate tofu in a mixture of tamari, sugar, ginger, and lemon juice for two hours. Heat oil in a skillet on medium heat. Add marinated tofu and cook for 10 minutes. Serve with brown rice.

GRAIN SALAD

¼ cup bulghur
1 cup boiling water
¼ cup wild rice
2 cups water
⅛ tsp. salt

¼ cup pecans

¼ cup celery, chopped fine

¼ cup mushroom cap slices

1 scallion, sliced thin

¼ cup parsley, minced

½ tsp. raw brown sugar

¼ cup cooking oil

1 tsp. fresh lemon or lime juice

½ cup shrimp, boiled and shelled, or ½ cup cut tofu for vegetarians

Salt and pepper to taste

A little fresh cilantro for decoration

Place bulghur in a bowl and add 1 cup boiling water. Cover and let sit for 2–3 hours. Drain and squeeze all excess moisture from the grain by hand and set aside. In another pot, bring wild rice and ⅛ tsp. salt to a boil in 2 cups of water. Cover and turn heat to medium low. Cook about 15 minutes. Drain and spread on a baking sheet to cool.

Preheat oven to 350°F. Put pecans on a cookie sheet and roast in the oven for 8 minutes. Remove, transfer to a plate, and let cool. Chop pecans coarsely and combine with rice and bulghur. Add celery, mushrooms, scallion, and parsley. In another bowl, mix together sugar, oil, lemon juice, shrimp or tofu, salt and pepper. Pour on top of the bulghur mixture. Garnish with cilantro.

GRANOLA

Dry Ingredients:

1 cup sunflower seeds

1 cup wheat germ

7 cups oats

4 cups crisped rice cereal

1 cup date pieces
1 cup almond pieces
1 cup coconut
1 cup sesame seeds

Wet Ingredients:
1 cup packed raw brown sugar
1 cup safflower oil
½ cup honey
1 17-oz. can apple sauce
1 tbsp. crushed orange peel
1 tbsp. real vanilla extract
1 tsp. cinnamon

Preheat oven to 350°F. In a large bowl mix together all dry ingredients. Combine wet ingredients at room temperature in another bowl, stirring until evenly mixed. Pour over mixture of dry ingredients. Mix together well and spread on a cookie tin, forming a layer 1½″ thick. Bake in the oven, checking regularly. When the top gets brown, turn ingredients over a few times. Do the same about three times until everything in the mixture gets nice and brown. Makes about 5 lbs. of granola. Great for breakfast or a snack.

SEAWEED WITH CABBAGE

1 cup hijiki seaweed
1 tsp. sesame oil
1 cup thinly sliced cabbage
1 medium carrot, sliced thin

Soak hijiki for 15 minutes. Drain well and save the water. Heat oil in a pan and sauté cabbage. Add carrot, hijiki, and the saved soaking water.

Simmer until tender. Season with soy sauce or tamari. Garnish with fresh cilantro or parsley and sesame seeds. Serve with brown rice.

SOYBEAN PUDDING

¼ cup syrup (brown rice, maple, or barley syrup)
3 cups soybean milk
1 bar agar agar

Warm soybean milk and add agar. Cook until melted. Add syrup and pour into small bowls. Let set until firm. Refrigerate for ½ hour. Add fruit slices on top for decoration if desired.

STEAMED ARTICHOKES

1 artichoke per person
Melted butter
Lemon juice or Artichoke Dip (see recipe under *Dressings and Sauces*).

Trim 1 to 2 inches off the top of each artichoke and all but ½ inch off the stem. Cut the tip ends off of the large outer leaves with scissors. Rinse the outer surfaces and let some pure water settle in the center of the leaves. Steam artichokes in a pan or double boiler for 20 to 35 minutes, depending on size. Remove from pan and let cool. Eat with Artichoke Dip, melted butter, or lemon juice.

STIR-FRIED BOK CHOY WITH BLACK MUSHROOMS

1 stalk bok choy, cut into ½" pieces
Soy sauce to taste
5 black mushrooms, soaked and cut into fourths
Cooking oil (olive, safflower, or sesame)

Add cooking oil to a heated skillet and sauté bok choy and black mushrooms. Add a dash of salt and soy sauce to taste. Cook for 5 minutes.

STIR-FRIED CHAYOTE AND CARROTS

2 chayote, peeled and cut into small pieces (or 1 bunch of broccoli)
1 carrot, cut into small strips
1 onion, chopped
2 tbsp. cooking oil
Soy sauce to taste

Sauté onion in oil in a heated skillet until fragrant. Add chayote and carrots and season with soy sauce. Simmer for 7–10 minutes. Serve with rice.

SWEET AND SOUR EGGPLANT

1 medium eggplant, peeled and cut into bite-sized pieces
1 medium onion, cut into small pieces
½ cup olive oil
Basil (optional)
1 tbsp. soy sauce
1 tsp. raw brown sugar
1 tbsp. vinegar

Mix together soy sauce, raw brown sugar, and vinegar. Set aside. In a small pan, heat oil and add onion and eggplant. Gently stir until eggplant is evenly cooked, soft, and tender. Add soy sauce, sugar and vinegar mixture. Sprinkle with basil if desired. Eat hot or cold. Excellent on brown rice.

TOFU AND BLACK MUSHROOMS

8 black mushrooms
1 lb. tofu
2 tbsp. soy sauce
1 tsp. cooking oil

Soak mushrooms for 10 minutes in water. Cut the stems off and discard. Cut tofu into 1-inch squares. In a heated skillet, add oil and sauté tofu and black mushrooms. Cover with a lid and lower heat for 10 minutes. Serve warm with rice. You may add vegetables (especially carrots, cauliflower or broccoli) to this recipe.

ZUCCHINI-EGGPLANT COMBINATION

1 lb. zucchini, cut into ⅛″ pieces
1 medium eggplant, peeled, quartered, and cut into ⅛″ pieces
2 tbsp. tamari
1 lb. tomatoes, peeled and chopped fine
1 tsp. basil
1 tsp. raw brown sugar
3 tbsp. cooking oil
Salt to taste

Heat 1 tbsp. cooking oil in a pot and sauté tomatoes, basil, and sugar. Cook for 10 minutes. In another pan, heat 2 tbsp. cooking oil and sauté zucchini and eggplant pieces. Season with tamari and stir until everything is evenly cooked. Add the cooked tomatoes and simmer for another 10 minutes. Serve over brown rice.

personal and home care

Supporting a Balanced State
in Daily Living

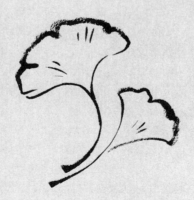

Cleansing

as you continue on toward health and vitality by transforming your dietary practices, you will also become more conscious of taking care of yourself in other aspects of your life. You can enhance your daily regime to promote and support your quest for greater health and for achieving a balanced state of being. As you know, what works well for one person may not work well for another. Feel free to make the necessary adjustments to these recommendations to suit your own lifestyle.

BATHING

Bathing is such a routine part of our personal care that we do not give it much thought. Yet it is a process that has very vitalizing effects on our system and energy. The tips below can help detoxify the body and make bathing a much more pleasurable and rejuvenating experience.

- Avoid bathing if you feel sick, if you are developing the symptoms of a cold, or if the weather is too damp. When sick or in a weak and vulnerable condition, the body needs to conserve every ounce of energy it has. Bathing drains some of your energy and may therefore contribute to a weakening of your body's defenses.

- When your hair is wet or damp, avoid exposure to air conditioning, drafts, and the wind. These can cause headaches and/or stiffness in the neck.

- Bathe with warm water and rinse with cold water. A cold water rinse will close the pores and "seal" the body's most vulnerable points of attack. It will also promote strong circulation.

- Once a week, after bathing, treat your body to a lemon shower. Scrub from head to toe with fresh lemons or limes. Allow the juice and pulp to remain on the skin for 10 minutes and rinse thoroughly. This rids the body of bacteria and negative energy. It will make you feel wonderful.

- Oil your body with coconut or olive oil three days after the lemon shower. Let it remain on the skin for 30 minutes before bathing and rinsing. This will enhance and protect the skin and give it a healthy glow.

HERBAL STEAM

Treating yourself to an occasional herbal steam bath is refreshing and highly recommended. It helps remove toxins and negative energy from your body. When you feel the flu or any other illness creeping up on you, an herbal steam may help revive your energies and ward off the illness. Follow the directions below for a wonderfully refreshing herbal steam.

Herbal Steam Recipe
- Bring approximately 6 quarts of water to a boil in a large pot. Add 2 stalks of lemon grass and 1 thumb-sized piece of fresh ginger and allow to steam.

- Place the pot on a board or a book on the floor and sit close to it. Completely cover yourself and the pot with one or two heavy blankets to retain the heat, allowing the herbal steam to induce perspiration. Use a chopstick to stir the water slowly as you sit. This will help release a steady flow of steam to make you perspire well.

- Remain under the blankets for at least 10 minutes.

- After removing the blankets, take a quick warm shower, put on warm clothes, and lie down for 30 minutes. Avoid any drafts.

The pot of herbs can be re-steamed for another member of the family. Do not use more than twice, however, since most of the essence of the herbs will have been steamed off by the end of the second usage.

INTERNAL CLEANSING

After decades of eating fast food, junk food, and poorly combined foods, it is vital for many people to consider a cleaning-out program. If you feel that you need to undertake such a program, be very careful not to take it to an extreme. If you are eating in a healthful way, cleansing would really be an integral part of your everyday diet. The Eastern way is to cleanse the blood every day by utilizing the natural properties of herbs, thoughtful preparation of food using a variety of cooking methods, and combining foods for balanced meals.

With this in mind, taking the attitude that you can quickly rid your body of the harmful effects of twenty years of junk food becomes ludicrous. As with everything else, each new adjustment you make to your eating and health habits should be undertaken in moderation. Have the understanding and attitude that you are changing your bad habits permanently, not just until you get well or lose weight.

Colonics

Recently, there has been a flood of information written about colonics. I have read much, done some research, and experimented with them myself. I have great respect for colonic therapy and feel that it has saved lives in numerous cases of advanced toxicity. But I do not believe, as many of my fellow practitioners do, that everyone, no matter who they are or what circumstances they are in, needs a colonic. There are no absolutes in life. Not everyone needs a colonic. It is important not to give a colonic to those whose health is fragile, weak, depleted, sick, or malnourished. On the other hand, those who have a strong constitution but are prone to constipation, may benefit from a colonic or enema once in a while.

Constipation is a big complaint among my patients, usually caused by poor diet. This condition should be monitored closely since it is dangerous to health. Toxic wastes must be able to eliminate daily to keep the body pure and clean. Constipation stops this process and allows toxins and poisons to back up to the brain through the blood stream. Chronic constipation is serious because it can lead to many other diseases. It is best to first consider the diet, lifestyle, and emotional inclinations of a person who is prone to constipation before deciding that a colonic is the best form of treatment.

Some cautions about treatment methods are also warranted. There are many people giving colonics, but few really know what to consider when applying this treatment. Important considerations include (1) the sanitary conditions of the treatment facility. It is imperative that all instruments be properly sterilized so that the anus does not become a receptacle for contagious diseases and viruses entering the body; (2) the method of massage applied to the abdomen as the trajectory of water goes into the body; (3) the amount of oxygen in the water; (4) the intensity of the yellow light shining into the abdomen to assist the mobilizing action of the intestine in elimination; (5) the gentleness, kindness, compassion, and honesty of the practitioner; and (6) the practitioner should be knowledgeable in advising the client what to do before and after receiving the colonic.

Enemas

If it is not convenient for you to receive a colonic or if you are too weak for the treatment, it can be helpful to give yourself an enema. Either one of the following formulas is suitable for this:

1. 1 quart warm water, 1 pinch of salt, juice of one lemon. Apply the whole quart of water. Stand up. Repeat with one quart of the same solution but using cold water.

   OR

2. 1 pinch of salt, 1 tsp. anise powder, 1 tsp. castor oil, ½ gallon warm water. Apply the whole solution.

A glass of ginger tea with honey will assure that your energy remains stable and undepleted following the enema. After an enema, you should avoid eating processed foods, those made with white flour, alcohol, soft drinks, dried foods, cigarettes, cheese, milk, and other dairy products.

Chicken, barley soup, vegetable soup, and steamed green vegetables such as okra, kale, broccoli, and watercress are recommended. These foods help strengthen the body and ensure that the intestine does not get blocked again.

Sometimes, after having an enema, you will not have a bowel movement the next day. Do not get discouraged. Just continue to eliminate bad foods and eat wholesome foods. Your body will regain its natural balance.

Fasting

The idea behind fasting is to slow your body rhythm down and allow it to rest. Gentle fasting is best to maintain balance in your system. Start by gradually working away from foods like coffee, chocolate, pastries, and other toxic foods so that when you decide to go on a more strict fast, your body will have had time to eliminate toxins that could cause severe discomfort.

For those who have never fasted before, start with a one-day fast every six months with seasonal fruit or soy milk. I have found soy milk to be best in my own experience. Later, you can progress to once a week for a few months and then a few days a week. Do not torture yourself to satisfy your ego. Your system will only be thrown off balance and you may make yourself sick.

In deciding when to fast, choose a day that does not require much physical labor and when you have the least exposure to radiation from TV screens. Resting on the beach or meditating are good activities. Take things slowly and in an appreciative manner. Fasting is a time for the body, mind, and spirit to rest in peace and harmony.

The best time of the year to fast is springtime, and it is best done with strawberries or tomatoes. In the summer, fast with watermelon, soy milk, or lemon juice. Use one lemon with one glass of water and one table-spoon of pure olive oil first thing in the morning. If the lemon juice mixture makes you feel weak, drink soy milk only for a while.

Carrot juice, lemon juice, mung bean sprouts, and alfalfa sprouts are all good for cleansing blood under certain conditions. Again, you must remain mindful of the state of your health at the time you are considering a fast and the best cleansing foods for your particular condition.

I do not recommend having sex while fasting. Sensual activity requires a lot of energy and is a stimulant, therefore it is contradictory to the fasting state. I also do not recommend fasting for those who have become weak or depleted.

Most important, plan to continue to live simply, cleanly, and with a loving attitude after fasting. It is not wise to fast and to then go back to bad habits. Your body will not appreciate it, and your spirit will not benefit from these extremes.

RESTING, MOVING, AND BREATHING

Your body and spirit need rest and relaxation to efficiently maintain functioning, to rejuvenate energy, and to digest the experiences of your life. Napping, conscious relaxation, and sleep are all vitally important in maintaining health and balance. Also essential to your balance are the ways you move and breathe. Proper motion and breathing help prevent stagnation, not only in our physical lives, but in our emotional, intellectual, and spiritual lives as well. Sitting in front of a television night after night is a sure way of becoming dull and losing your energy and creativity.

NAPPING

Napping is an activity that can help reduce stress and increase well-being by renewing energy. In China and many oriental countries, a two-hour break is usually taken after the noon meal, from noon until 2:00 PM or from 1:00 PM until 3:00 PM. It is believed that this practice aids digestion, since a sleeping body is in a high state of anabolism (constructive metabolism). More digestive juices are produced, wastes are more rapidly removed by the blood cells, and fresh blood cells are more efficiently pumped to the skeletal muscles.

Some researchers believe that naps stimulate your creative processes because the brain is actually twice as active during sleep, analyzing the events that have taken place in your waking hours. At the very least, naps can supplement any lack of nighttime sleep and thus keep your body in a better balance all day.

Keep your naps as regular as possible. Start and finish at the same time each day. If you are in a situation where napping is impossible, try at least to take a little time to relax. Read a magazine, listen to music, or take a short stroll in a park; any of these activities will refresh your energy and make the rest of your day enjoyable.

SLEEPING

We spend approximately one-third of our lives sleeping, therefore it merits due consideration as an important part of our daily life. Not only do our sleeping hours re-energize us for the next day, but our bodies undergo a cleansing process at the same time. Recognize the need for good sound sleep and assist your body in performing this important function. The following suggestions should prove helpful to you.

- Always try to sleep with your head to the north. This will assist the rest and cleansing process by aligning your magnetic polarity to that of the earth as a whole.

- Sleep on your back or your right side to keep pressure off your most vital organs. This will help prevent illness late in life.

- Support your spine and maintain your posture during sleep with a high-quality firm mattress. If you have backaches, support the weight of your legs by placing a pillow under your knees when lying on your back, or put your thighs perpendicular to the rest of your body when lying on your right side.

- Sleep for a sufficient amount of time each night to provide a deep rest for your body—usually seven or eight hours. Rest in a quiet, peaceful setting that provides adequate fresh air and ventilation.

- Walk barefoot in the grass for five or ten minutes before retiring to allow quicker dissipation of pent-up energy and to relieve the tensions of a stressful day. A warm shower before bedtime will also help.

- Always sleep with some type of covering over your lower abdomen or "hara." This is considered the "sea of Qi" or the central storage place of your vital energy in oriental medicine. Keeping this area covered will protect your essence, which in turn will make you less vulnerable to disease and sickness. A sheet, shirt, pajamas, or anything made of one hundred percent cotton is recommended.

MOVING

We often judge someone's general personality from their movements and appearance. Realizing this, move and act as you truly wish to be perceived. If you seek to be balanced and centered, concentrate on moving with purpose. Walk and act positively; do not sit too much, and be sure to stretch from time to time. Practicing moving with harmony, gracefulness, and purpose will assist you in the attainment of your goal of inner balance. Consider learning and practicing Tai Qi Ch'uan or Qi Kung. These are forms of Oriental exercise that tone the outer and inner body by combining movement with proper breathing techniques.

BREATHING

Through breath, the body takes in the essence of life. Few people, however, breathe in a way that most effectively draws the energy through their systems. The breath should be long and slow and should fill the lower abdomen. It should continually draw the energy and life essence into the solar plexus, the hara or "sea of Qi."

Traditional Chinese medicine teaches that in a fetus the Qi moves down from within the mother as she breathes and enters the fetus through the umbilical cord. From there it goes to the head and down the front of the face to the tongue, throat, and on to the vital organs. The energy finally settles behind the navel in the lower abdomen, where energy is stored in each of us.

Sometime after birth, for some unknown reason, most of us lose the natural instinct to breathe into the abdomen and begin to breathe into our lungs. This way of breathing denies us the full potential in the energy of each breath. It requires conscious effort to breathe correctly; learning the right way to breathe will take some time. Watch a baby to help you learn the correct way. The following suggestions will also help you.

- Start by lying on your back and letting your arms, legs, and entire body relax. Wear clothing that does not constrict your body, especially around the waist.

- Place the tip of your tongue on the roof of your mouth just behind your upper front teeth, and let your mouth close until your teeth gently touch each other. This connects the two most important meridians in the body (the govern vessel and the conception vessel), making a long circuit through which the Qi will flow as you take each breath. It is said that the fetus always has the tip of its tongue touching the roof of its mouth while in its mother's womb, completing the same circuit.

- Close your eyes, relax, and concentrate on your hara, one inch below your navel.

- Take a long, slow, deep breath through your nose, filling the abdomen with air. At the end of the breath, stop and hold the air for just a few seconds, then exhale through your nose and mouth. Review the illustrations below to assist you.

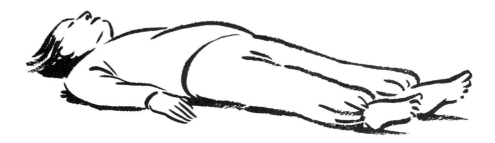

CORRECT INHALATION

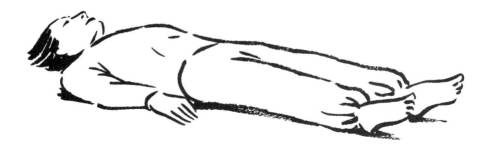

CORRECT EXHALATION

- When you first start practicing, place a medium-weight book directly over your navel to help you get in touch with the proper movement. With concentration, breathe so that your abdomen, along with the book, rises and gently falls with each breath.

- Practice on an empty stomach (three hours after meals or first thing in the morning). Always try to keep your tongue on the roof of your mouth. This will enable your Qi to flow through a greater length of your body and will provide you with more energy.

- After you are comfortable with this technique let your heart use its powerful energy to transform negative emotions to love, compassion, joy, and happiness. Use your breathing to dissolve tensions on the inhale and release positive loving energies into the world on the exhale.

- Remember not to breathe too fast or too slow. Breathing too fast will not be as cleansing or refreshing and you may hyperventilate. Breathing too slowly may put you to sleep, which is not usually the desired result. Breathe with rhythm and at a natural, smooth, and comfortable pace.

This is an excellent way to relax, reduce stress, balance and stimulate your energy. It can be done at work or almost anywhere. Your goal should be to learn to breathe naturally into your abdomen on a constant basis and to keep circulating your energy throughout your day.

Although breathing appears last in the personal care section, I believe it is the first and most important step in becoming healthier. It assists the circulatory system, encouraging blood to flow more freely on the inhale, while providing for the detoxification of the body on the exhale.

In fact, in their eagerness to get well, many of my patients ask me what they can do to help accelerate their healing. My most immediate response is usually to encourage much more attention to breathing. Breathing is our first and most important connection to God. Conscious breathing techniques move you away from short quick breaths; conscious breathing can mean the difference between living to survive and living to create. Don't let busy schedules distract you from deep breathing on a regular basis.

Remember that breath is a major contributor to the process of God realization. The manifestation of the living God within will not occur if we do not become mindful of the promise of eternal life that comes with each conscious breath we take.

THE HOME: HARMONIZING YOUR ENVIRONMENT

Many of us think of home as a place of warmth and comfort, a safe haven where we are nurtured and can retreat from the hazards of the outside world. Today, this is not necessarily true—the contemporary American home can be an unhealthy place. Studies done by the Environmental Protection Agency indicate that the concentration of dangerous air pollutants can be up to one hundred times greater inside your home than outside. A careful assessment of your living space, from your kitchen to your bedrooms and bathroom, will probably reveal the presence of many products containing chemically volatile substances that can have an insidious detrimental effect on your health.

PLASTICS AND SYNTHETICS

Plastics in household items manufactured from polyvinyl chloride present particularly pervasive health hazards in the home. They continuously release vapors of carcinogenic vinyl chloride. Seemingly harmless items like vinyl flooring, upholstery fabrics, plastic containers, raincoats, shower curtains, and many toys may all be emitting this vapor. The hazard is especially acute with new items that are off-gassing. You can reduce the hazardous impact of some of these items by replacing them with wooden boxes, glass bottles, natural baskets, cotton products, and wooden toys.

Another hazardous product used in home construction and increasingly in furniture is particleboard. Particle board is made of sawdust and small wood chips which are pressed together and preserved with formaldehyde, a suspected carcinogen. Formaldehyde vapor is released into the home atmosphere in large quantities by particleboard. To protect yourself from the chemical cloud of formaldehyde fumes, you can seal items made of particleboard by painting on a vapor barrier finish.

CLEANING PRODUCTS AND PESTICIDES

The products we use for household cleaning and eliminating insect pests are also big environmental culprits in the home. They are full of chemicals that pose health hazards when inhaled over long periods of time. Many can be at the root of chronic respiratory, skin, sinus, and nervous problems. Consider using the alternative cleaners and pesticides listed below.

Alternative Household Cleaners

- General Household Cleaning Abrasives: Use baking soda, lemon juice, white vinegar, borax, natural soap, or trisodium phosphate (TSP) for household cleaning.

- Gentle Household Cleaner: 1 teaspoon TSP, liquid soap or borax, and 1 quart of warm water. If cleaning grease, add vinegar or lemon. Mix together and put in a spray bottle.

- Furniture Polish: Mix together 1 teaspoon of olive oil, 1 teaspoon of brandy, 1 teaspoon of water, and the juice of 1 lemon. Make fresh each time.

Alternative Home Pesticides

- Ants: Find out where they are coming from and sprinkle dried mint leaves. They will go away.

- Beetles: Place a bay leaf in each grain container or store containers in the refrigerator to keep them cool and fresh. If you have large amounts of grain to store, expose the grain to the sun four or five hours once a month so it can reap the benefits of the sun's energy and stay fresh and bug-free.

- Cockroaches: Mix together equal parts of baking soda and powdered sugar and spread around infested area. Repeat several times at two-week intervals until the roaches are gone.

- Flies: Scratch the skin of an orange or tangerine and let it sit out. The citrus oil released from the rind will repel flies.

ALUMINUM

Aluminum is another well-known source of toxicity. It can accumulate in various human tissues, such as the brain, liver, and bone tissues, and may have an adverse affect on memory in adults. It may also be a factor in learning disabilities and behavioral problems in younger people. With this in mind, try to avoid products that contain aluminum, such as some toothpastes, chewing gum, cosmetics, most antiperspirants, many over-the-counter pharmaceuticals, industrial abrasives, and paints. Some of the deleterious effects of aluminum can be reduced by supplementing the diet with zinc, magnesium, manganese, and vitamin C. Consult your acupuncturist or family physician before taking these.

TAP WATER

The tap water we use on a daily basis is nowadays, unfortunately, always suspect as a source of pollutants. Studies have shown that a good percentage of our exposure to water pollutants comes from absorption through the skin while bathing. Many of us start the day with a shower to freshen up and wake up. To protect yourself from water pollutants, you can install an activated carbon filter. It can be installed to either filter the water in the whole house or to filter just at the shower head. These attachments are very effective and inexpensive.

inner balance

Meditation and Growth

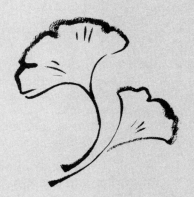

MEDITATION

*i*n today's stressful world, diseases often stem from such emotions as anxiety, fear, and anger. These emotional states make it difficult to stay in harmony with the universe. Taking time each day to practice meditation is not only highly recommended but actually becomes necessary to our well-being. Meditation is a potent healing tool. It gives us time to release tensions, reflect on the daily events of our lives, and renew our energies to live each day with clarity and enthusiasm.

Meditation does not involve expensive equipment and therefore does not add to the complexities of life. The following three items are its simple requirements:

1. A certain posture of the body

2. A certain breathing technique

3. A certain attitude of the mind

POSTURE

Sit on a cushion with your legs comfortably crossed. Sit so that your knees are lower than your hips and your spine is erect. If you are a little stiff, you may need to use two pillows or you can sit on a chair with your feet flat on the floor.

Tip your pelvis slightly forward and relax your abdomen. Draw your chin gently down and inward. Rest your left hand in your right with palms up; join the tips of your thumbs to form an oval shape. Relax your shoulders. Try to keep the tip of your tongue resting lightly at the top of your palate, behind your front teeth.

If you feel sleepy or lethargic, keep your eyes slightly open and direct your gaze downward, looking at nothing in particular. If you feel restless or overly active, close your eyes. Focus your mind on the rising and falling of your abdomen; your thoughts should be in harmony with your breath.

BREATHING

As you sit in meditation, follow the flow of your breath; it is the vital link between your body and the cosmic energy. In the act of breathing, energy is transmitted to all the cells of the body. The breath serves as a medium for dispelling negative energy and recharging the body with fresh positive energy.

Breathing assists meditative activity by strengthening the body's Qi, our vital force, the attentive energy of our non-thinking, intuitive, deep awareness. Deep breathing enables us to make this awareness strong and steady.

Breathe in a slow natural rhythm. Exhale for as long as possible with your attention focused on the flow of the breath. Let your inhalation come naturally. Do not force the breath; it should be slow, smooth, steady, and comfortable.

Let your thoughts and mental images pass like clouds in the sky while you concentrate on your breath. Think with your body; think without thinking, with all contradictions transcended. The sustained practice of meditation causes your brain to be flooded with the same alpha waves that are found in deep sleep. Putting yourself in this state of relaxation while practicing the technique of prolonged exhalation gives your brain a rest and enables your body to eliminate nervous tension.

Sit in meditation for about twenty minutes. It is best to do this regularly for twenty minutes after you rise and another twenty minutes before you go to bed.

ATTITUDE OF THE MIND

Health is as much a state of mind as it is a physical state. Without the determination and commitment of the mind, attaining good health is an elusive goal. The brain is a miraculous instrument. Put to full use, its immense power, teamed with the body, can lead to tremendous feats of accomplishment. Left unused, it becomes stagnant and wastes away.

Your life is but a drop of water in the sea of time. Only you can decide whether to accomplish a lot or a little. Make use of the abilities and opportunities at hand and live life to its fullest potential. The following suggestions should help you:

- Keep positive and loving thoughts in your mind. Be kind and humble to yourself as well as to others. Develop and utilize compassion, one of the most admirable traits a human can possess.

- Read good books on a variety of subjects. These will be a source of inspiration to you and will propel your growth.

- Be devoted to yourself. This is a deeper vow than commitment and will assure that you stay on the right track, always moving forward, always growing.

To illustrate the power of attitude, we can use the example of waiting for a friend who is late for a meeting. On the one hand, you could allow the situation to create stress by feeling angry or victimized. This would be detrimental to your health. On the other hand, you could take the attitude that you have an opportunity to spend a few minutes relaxing and refreshing yourself. You could focus your attention on the solar plexus and open up to the power of its energy. Try doing this simple exercise, accompanied by deep breathing, to convince you of its benefits. It will increase your vitality for the rest of the day and reinforce your sense of flow with the events happening around you. It will also encourage your acceptance of what life brings to you.

The entire process of living a prosperous and healthy life can be summarized in a brief but powerful sentence:

Before you can conquer the large universe,
you must first conquer the small universe.

The large universe is the one in which we all exist; the one in which we strive to attain our goals or leave our mark. The small universe is the one existing within each of us; the one in which we struggle to be balanced and wise. The large universe can never be conquered without having first conquered the small one. Conquer your small universe and the large universe is at your command. Attempt to by-pass the small universe and the large universe becomes your enemy.

Good health is more than a sense of physical well-being. It is more than the absence of disease. Good health includes a quality of being that emanates from the spiritual and mental levels as well as the physical. It includes the experience of a clear mind, keen emotional balance, intuitive perception, and a spiritual understanding which allows you to feel your connection with all others and with the universe. In balanced harmony you flow gracefully with life, responding to all circumstances with accuracy and impeccability.

Life is a learning process, and we are here to grow. I encourage you to use this manual as a stepping stone along the simple path to health and happiness. With practice and patience, you will continue to move forward.

ABOUT THE AUTHOR

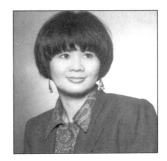

born in South Vietnam, Dr. Le arrived in the United States in 1979 after fleeing Vietnam as a refugee with several thousand other "boat people." Healing is her second nature and was the vital force that helped her overcome all the trials and obstacles during her first few years in the new country. In five short years she reestablished her profession, first as a licensed practical nurse, then as a certified acupuncturist and a Ph. D. in Traditional Chinese Medicine. She accomplished this while supporting her two children, overcoming the language barrier, and coping with an unending homesickness for her large family that she had to leave behind.

Kim Le is a third generation Chinese acupuncturist who trained as such in Vietnam and China. She has worked extensively in American hospitals and clinics. She is a member of the American Society of Acupuncturists of Pennsylvania, and the National Commission for the Certification of Acupuncturists and Herbalists (NCCA). She has taught Chinese medicine at local universities, health care institutes in the United States, and abroad.

In 1980 she founded the Kim Le Clinic and presently practices in Colorado Springs, Colorado. The Kim Le Clinic provides traditional Chinese medicine treatments which include acupuncture, nutritional counseling, lifestyle consultations, and meditation instruction. Dr. Le's books include: *Path of Compassion* (1994), *In Search of the "I"* (1993), *Compassionate Eating* (1991), and *A Theory of Preventative and Remedial Nutrition for Good Health* (1985).